Satiated: Finding salvation in sugar, sex and surfing

A memoir

By Natasha Black

With special thanks to MRG for coaching me, believing in me and setting me straight when I needed it. To CL for pushing me to do this. To TE for listening to me hash all this out and living parts of it with me.

Introduction

PART I - Sugar

PART II - Surf

Introduction

My heart raced. I laid my index and middle finger to my neck, timing my pulse. *I seriously need to calm down*, I thought, knowing that it wouldn't happen. For an hour, I'd surveyed the breaking waves, judging where I wanted to enter the water, what line I wanted to take on the paddle out, where I wanted to sit among the other surfers. Most of all, I'd surveyed my inner self, and whether I had what it would take to ride one of those giants.

I was about to do something surfers only dream of doing. I was about to paddle out at one of the most famous big wave surfing arenas in the world. Many had lost their lives here. This is where boys become men. This is where women become warriors. Would this be where I would finally find what it was I was after? I sat and watched. Was it my ego that said I was good enough? My lack of self-confidence that said I wasn't?

I gathered my surf tools and walked down to the beach. Under one arm I carried a ten-foot surfboard shaped for big waves, known as a "gun". My free hand clutched an extra thick surfboard leash, made specifically not to break in heavy conditions, and an impact vest designed to help with floatation and in absorbing some of the thousands of foot-pounds of pressure created by house-sized waves crashing over my body.
I carried the vest in my hand rather than wearing it because I knew there were surf paparazzi swarming the beach. I knew I was the only woman who would be surfing and I knew I looked much cuter in a hot pink bikini than I did with a padded vest that made me look like a linebacker. I passed by a young family on the beach as I headed to the entry zone. The mother saw me. Nudging her young daughter, she whispered,

"Look, she is going to charge it out there!" Her words gave me chills. That one stroke of ego at once calmed and inspired me with an even bigger reason to do what I was about to do.

How big can I get? How much can I achieve? What will it take for people to know me? How many risks will I take and how much of my life will I give to receiving recognition?

Every time my ego steps out of the shadows and I am honest enough with myself to recognize it, I am sent into a panic. *What if they don't like me? What if they see through my act the same way I am now seeing through it? What if they have been seeing through it all along and laughing at me behind my back?*

I left the island just a few days after that first paddle out at Waimea Bay. It would almost be a year before I had the chance to, once again, surf the iconic behemoth. In that year, I would surf some of the world's heaviest surf, daily, pushing myself, challenging limits, defying fears, and accepting my physical punishments for each mistake with open arms along the way.

The next time I had the opportunity to surf Wiamea again it was the beginning of the winter season on the North Shore of Oahu. I saw the set coming. Several seconds would pass before it arrived at my place in the line-up. One of the guys who sat a bit deeper than me angled his head slightly and lifted his chin to give me *that* look: "This one is yours," he confirmed with his eyes. I had now been around this wave and these surfers long enough to have earned a few head nod's of respect like this one from a few of the guys. When an elder in the surf gives you a wave, you have to go, even if you'd rather stay safely outside of the take-off zone. This was a serious wave and that look had committed me whether I liked it or not. My mind geared into overdrive and dissolved into complete nothingness, all at once. Conscious thought was too slow a tool for the set that rose toward me. Muscle memory assumed control. My gaze narrowed, targeting the spot I would need to reach in order to catch the incoming wave. My highly trained breathing mirrored my strokes. My body entered a state of deep play with the ocean.

Within moments, the wave would be upon me. I had just seconds to reach the ideal take-off spot. I could hear the wave coming, though it made no sound. The face of the wave mounted and towered taller than a house. I felt myself pulled backward and up. Big waves like this create their own weather. Suddenly, I raced straight into the face of a tropical storm. I dug deeper, my body exerting maximum effort and maximum poise without a thought. The speed of my board increased. Now I was traveling as fast as the wave. I peered over the ledge of a twenty-five-foot drop into deep blue. It looked impossible to make. The wave face was nearly vertical and quickly becoming concave. But my experience told me it was indeed makeable. An intentional thought broke through my silent communion with the wave: *trust yourself, trust your equipment, trust your experience.*

That feeling of my feet landing in the right place, the fins catching, just the pointed "pin" of the tail penetrating the water's surface, my weight perfectly balanced over the surface chop -- the sudden knowing that I nailed the drop -- induces an inexplicable euphoria. I am catapulted into a more *real* level of reality. At that moment, I had no worry over the future and no regret of the past. That present moment is so electrifying that thoughts of the outside world are impossible. The verbal centers of the brain are deactivated because they are useless in that space. A new form of knowing fills my body. Time is irrelevant. There is the briefest pause in the endless suffering that is my life. I am okay.

Until a split second later. To make my bottom turn, I looked to my right and was startled by a flash of red. A woman in a red bathing suit--I knew her, but only from magazines--had "dropped in" on me. Dropping in is surfer-speak for cutting in front of another surfer, impeding their line of progress. The wise choice would have been for me to lean moderately into my inside rail, make a wide-bottom turn, and avoid her. But in my inexperience I panicked. Questions of worthiness paralyzed me. I didn't deserve to be out there, I didn't deserve to take up space on that wave. She was the pro, the local, I was nobody. Instead of turning toward her, I continued straight. My line of progress now mirrored the line of the cascading lip behind me. Instead of outrunning it, I was about to be hit in the back by an avalanche. I placed all my weight on my back foot. I braced for the lip to explode behind me.

What proceeded was a scene familiar from many action movies. A bomb explodes in a building, bodies fly out. The lip of the wave exploded into my back. My body flew several feet through the air, curved into a scorpion's arc. I went under, and the water's seemingly infinite strength pinned me there. I was underwater for what seemed like ages. My trained mind purposely emptied. This was no time for thinking. Out here, panic was equivalent to death. I calmly waited until I felt the power dissipated and kicked my way to the surface. But I barely registered the hold-down as sharp pain seared through my lower back. I had already been nursing a moderate back injury from months ago. It was getting worse with every server wipeout I had, which were many. I knew what had just happened to my body even before I lost bladder control, a telltale sign of spinal nerve damage. Though I refused to admit it, I already knew what an MRI would tell me a few weeks later: my entire lumbar spine had been severely damaged.

On the day I got my MRI results, I showed them to a surfer friend who was also a doctor for the World Surf League. He was known to be at Sunset Beach around the time of sunset each evening. I found him in his usual spot. I offered him the folded paper. Taking a seat, he donned his reading glasses. He inspected the dense medical language for several careful minutes while I wrung my hands and pretended to enjoy the spectrum of purples and pinks that now filled the sky. He removed his glasses. Then he looked up and spoke.

"Well, you have a lot of work ahead of you, kiddo. You will surf again, maybe in a year. I know your dream is to be a competitive big wave surfer. And I know how hard you've been working for it. But this changes everything. I would forget ever surfing big waves again."

The tears I had been holding back all day surged forth, all at once.

I walked the bike path north, from Sunset Beach to my studio apartment at Velzyland. I made no attempt to control my crying. I just pulled my hoodie over my head and wept as I walked. Big wave surfing was everything to me. It was the only thing big enough to take away the pain of it all. It told me who I was, it permitted me to be as big as I was. It was my identity. What was I without my body?

I surfed big waves in order to access the extremes of human experience, and I was having one, sure enough. The pain reached a depth I had only known twice before: once, when the love of my life disappeared in front of my eyes; and once, when an inner voice told me I would lose my perfect body in order to regain my spirit.

I knew at that moment that recovery would take the best of me. It would take more of me than I currently had to give. I knew that overcoming this obstacle, just like previous ones, would bring me to a place I didn't yet know existed, but a place I desperately needed to go. My body was in this state for a reason. In order to heal I would have to discover that reason. To what depth could I dive? What dark places would I travel?

As I stood in front of the mirrored wall at my first physical therapy appointment, I heard the words of my mother coming out of the doctor's mouth. "Straighten out your feet Natasha." In my mind, I was instantly transported to being nine years old and my mother was once again criticizing the way I walked, the way I was.

"When you let your feet collapse like that your knees knock inward and it results in hip rotation." The doctor continued. "This movement pattern, which you've likely had since childhood, is putting too much extension into your lumbar spine making it the weakest link in your body. If you ever want to return to surfing we have to correct the way you move in this world."

I lifted the arches in my feet and pressed my big toe downwards. As my feet straightened out, so did my knees and hips. This maneuver shifted my lower back out of extension and into a neutral position. Suddenly, all the pain in my lower back switched to a dull roar. My mother had been yelling at me to straighten out my feet since I was nine. And now it all made sense.

Something clicked. Suddenly, I knew for sure several things that had previously been a mystery.
I understood that in order to truly heal I would need to completely remake myself. I would need to deconstruct and to slow down to the point where I could focus on details as small as my big toe and as large as shame.

Next, I realized that healing my body was going to utterly deplete me. I would have to turn into the primordial soup found inside a chrysalis if I was ever to emerge as something functional.

Lastly, I realized that my mother had always loved me the best she knew how.

My process of healing was about more than returning my physical body to the state it was in before a wave exploded in my back. Behind that wave was a nine-year-old version of me who needed to relearn who she was.

Welcome to recovery.

PART I – Sugar

Chapter 1: Fundamentalism

"The first thing is your body. The body is your base...it is where you are grounded. To make you antagonistic toward the body is to destroy you...to make you miserable, to create hell."
-Osho

I was born into a white, religious, middle-class family. I'm the granddaughter of a farmer and a Detroit union auto laborer. My parents are still married to this day. We lived in a nice house. We took a vacation every year. My siblings and I, all five of us, had a car to drive upon turning sixteen. Despite her exhausting work homeschooling us, maintaining the household, and helping her own parents run their farm, my mom never brought home a paycheck. Dad was a hard worker, a dedicated father, a loving husband, and a good provider. There is no such thing as a perfect, or even normal, childhood, but mine was rather unremarkable.
My parents were doing what they thought was the best when they took my siblings and me to church at least three times per week. Singing, "Jesus loves me, this I know, for the Bible tells me so," practically from the womb taught me that, surely if the Bible said it, then it was true. I was indoctrinated to believe that the Bible, and more specifically the way my church interpreted the Bible, was the ultimate authority in all matters. It seemed perfectly normal when we were rewarded with plastic trinkets for memorizing Bible verses. When we grew too old for plastic prizes, my parents enrolled us on the Bible quiz team and paid us $1 per correct answer. No one thought it out of the ordinary, least of all me, when I memorized over half the New Testament by age sixteen. I did it because I wanted to win competitions. I wanted the trophy and the love I hoped would come with it. I was awarded MVQ (Most Valuable Quizzer) four years in a row.

By homeschooling us, my parents were able to keep me and my siblings in a controlled environment. We attended a homeschool co-op, which met once per week. Nearly all of the families involved in this co-op were homeschooling their children for the same reasons as my parents: to protect us from "worldly influences." To ensure against exposure to foreign ideas, all students had to write their "testimony," a statement of belief in the Bible and swearing to have accepted Jesus as their Savior.

I have so many memories from those co-op meetings. Like when they forbade us from wearing logos (like the Mickey Mouse T-shirts worn by some students). Parents took issue because Disney hires "the gays." Then there was "Prim," which is what we had to call our dancing-free prom. Because dancing leads to… well, ya know (I wasn't allowed to use the "s word," so I'll just let you use your imagination). I was lucky that I was flat-chested. I remember the fate of some of my friends when they showed up in their fancy formal gowns with a sliver of cleavage showing. They were handed duct tape and forced to tape over their indecency if they wanted to participate in the festivities. Then there was the speech and debate event where several moms complained that my skirt wasn't long enough. I was forced into a room with a male teacher and another female student, where we girls had to prove our skirts passed the dress code. Being skilled debaters, we pulled out the written dress code and showed the man that the official policy was skirts "at" the knee rather than "below" the knee. We were sent away with a warning not to wear the same clothing the following day or else we would have to forfeit the competition. It was explained that girls like us were the cause of many sins committed by older men. It never occurred to me that this was creepy. Instead, I felt like I had done something wrong.

One summer, my church youth group took a trip to learn and

practice apologetics. For several days, we studied how to use scripture and logic to win an argument with a "non-believer." Then they sent us out in pairs to the streets of Chicago to practice what we had learned. For two days, my partner and I walked up to complete strangers and asked them if they believed in Jesus. If they did not, we argued with them until they got mad and left us, or until we converted them. We were instructed to keep a tally of the converts. At the end of the day, we joined up with the other thousands of teens who had also been out witnessing, and we all shared our tallies. We were instructed to scream and cheer when the number of converts came on the big screen. Like the angels in heaven, we were to rejoice over lost souls coming home.

Church and the homeschool co-op were my life. I played guitar in the church praise band. I volunteered in the church nursery. I was captain of the Bible quiz team. Even the sports teams I played on were homeschool teams. I can't remember meeting any non-white or gay people. I'm not sure I knew any Democrats, although I do remember my mom hesitating to let me hang around Shannon because her parents voted for Bill Clinton.

I had faith. I scrupulously followed the instructions of my pastor and my youth leader. I kept unfailingly to my daily "devotional" time of prayer, and I studied scripture with intensity. I never smoked, drank, or did more than kiss a boy until well after high school. But, somehow, it never seemed enough. I never seemed enough.

I was the picture-perfect model for a late 20th-century evangelical teen. With all the good and ugly that comes along with that. Evangelical Christianity hangs on one haunting doctrine — the doctrine of never-good-enough, or "Original Sin." I was raised in a United Brethren church. In the statement of doctrine on the United Brethren church's official website (at the time of publication), this same concept is defined as "*Depravity*":

> **All persons are born...with an inherent tendency toward evil.** *This depravity has negatively affected and **is operative in every faculty of one's being**. Each person, because of the inherited depravity, when confronted by the world, the flesh and the devil, will follow the sinful nature, **deliberately choosing to ratify sin**, and thus assumes the **guilt** and **condemnation** belonging to a sinner.*

So that was that. I was a sinner, a bad person, right off the bat. I never even had a chance. But there was one way out. And that way was to follow the teachings of the church. The first of which was to deny the body. All desires of the flesh are evil. In order to overcome my depravity, I must deny myself.

My dad was the hardest working man I knew. My dad's father was a real hard-ass. The only thing I really remember about him is how he always made my dad feel like a piece of shit for the way he ran the family business. Nothing was ever good enough for Grandpa Ray. As a result, my dad worked endlessly. What my dad was able to do as a small business owner blows my mind. Providing for five hungry kids and allowing my mom to stay at home with us, he still found time to teach us to change the oil in our cars, how to shoot layups, how to bait a hook, and how to skin a buck, all without a single complaint. Not one. Not ever. I learned from my dad that hard work is all that matters. If you work as many hours per week as a human can reasonably sustain, then you can be squarely middle-class, comfortable, and safe. He modeled flawlessly that the body and its desires should be ignored; after all, there is always more work to be done. Last Christmas, my father ended up in the ER three times in one week, with blood pressure off the charts. Even though his body has urged him to slow down, he continues to ignore those evil desires of the flesh.

My mom could run a country. She is a real-life "Proverbs 31 woman." The oldest of three, she grew up on a farm with a father who always expected more out of her. She was a straight-A student, the main cook in the household by age nine, and milked the cows every day. Her father grew up with a shithead alcoholic for a dad. In turn, my grandfather had learned never to express his emotions. Instead, he unintentionally made my mom feel like she needed to do more to earn his love. These days, my mom remodels bathrooms, lays tile, leads a Bible study, drives a tractor, runs the homeschool co-op we used to attend, serves on the board of directors at church, constantly babysits grandkids, throws pool parties, and has the entire family--eighteen of us--over for Sunday dinner every week. She is never idle. She never rests. And she also suffers from bleeding ulcers, insomnia, and high levels of anxiety. But this is my story, not hers.

I too understood on a cellular level that I would never be good enough. My body was flawed. My mind was its master. A good Christian would have to learn to control the desires of the flesh. They told me that my love for Jesus, my gratitude for what he did for me on the cross, would be enough that I would want to follow his commands and the desires of the flesh would melt away. But something wasn't adding up. I tried to love Jesus. But I still wanted to do things I wasn't supposed to. I didn't want to be nice all the time. I didn't feel like being quiet as good little girls should be. Something was wrong with me. I followed the formula but it wasn't working. I was a "wretch," as the hymn "*Amazing Grace*" puts it.

I once heard that God uses certain humans to cry his own tears. From the womb, powerful emotions have been my dark gift.

Feeling uncomfortably deeply has always been a part of my life. As a child, I constantly embarrassed myself at the dinner table with emotional outbursts. My mother always said that I should be a drama queen. I didn't understand what that meant. I wasn't acting. My brothers would roll their eyes and mock me, "Here come Natasha's elephant tears again!" I'd often flee the dinner table and run to my room, hot tears pouring down my face.

Inherited from a past life or imprinted within the cradle by a hurting mother, heavy pain is woven into my DNA. Some kids are just happy. I wasn't.

At the age of seven, the bleak gifts of depression and anxiety came rushing into my life. Alone in the basement of my parents' house, I was feeling sad and lonely. By then, I had already accepted such feelings as normal for me. It became too much to bear. Pain overwhelmed me, surging through the room in a rush of energy. I began to vibrate, my very cells shaking. The sensation was powerful and tangible. I was overcome and wept uncontrollably. One of my brothers found me and attempted, through my heaving sobs, to extract an explanation of what had happened.

I struggled intensely to make sense of the event. I didn't want to worry anyone. I looked for a way to make light of the terrifying episode. Synapses fired, electrical currents lashing through my young brain, seeking familiar pathways to set in context this other-worldly event. The currents landed on the religious narrative I had consumed each week in children's church. I pieced together the best explanation I could. I told my brother that Jesus had come into my heart and, at that moment, I had been born again. Indeed, I had been. From that point forward, depression and anxiety would be my constant companions.

It feels like a mini hurricane right underneath my sternum. It forms a whirlpool of hot stinging energy. It screams at me, "Do something! You are wasting your one shot at life!" It picks me up, it moves me -- to check my phone, to reach my hand into a bag of chips, to send a text, to check my email, to revisit the kitchen. I try to control it -- I go surf, I go shop, I go for a run, sometimes I smoke or drink or have sex, but most of the time I eat.

Even as a child, I knew something wasn't right. I had all the faith you could ask for. I excelled in every endeavor, from sports to academics to performing arts. None of it was enough. The predictions of well-meaning adults rang painfully in my ears:

"You are going to change the world!"
"You are unique."
"You are going places with your life."

Even the Bible haunted me. "I can do all things through Christ who strengthens me." Philippians 4:13. The most ear-piercing words of all came from my mother. "Natasha, you are so bound and determined. You can do anything you set your mind to." I had just this one shot to get it right, and afterward, final judgment. Time was limited. Every moment mattered. I mustn't sit idle, I mustn't waste time on frivolities like leisure and recreation, I must be productive, I must achieve something, and I must improve my sinful self!

It was a backpack full of bricks. I couldn't breathe under the weight of its responsibility. The terror that I might be infinitely powerful yet somehow choose the wrong path or not work hard enough for it...that I might let the whole world down. It created intense pressure on my chest. Anxiety plagued me. If I wasn't producing something at every

moment for the Kingdom, then I was wasting time. I couldn't
sleep at night. I was unable to get up in the morning. I lay
awake, writing in my journal about all the ways I was falling
short and all my plans to fix my flaws. I prayed to God to fix
me since I was obviously screwing everything up.

From the age of 10, I filled journals with melancholy poems. I
wrote prayers to God, asking him to change me, to make me
better. "Reveal your path for me," I would scribble. "I don't
want to follow my will, but your will for my life." My
despondent writing ranged from wondering why I didn't
have any friends to lists of all the reasons my parents surely
hated me, and how I hated them back. Honestly, I think they
did and also that they loved me. I'm not a parent yet, but I'm
pretty sure it's normal for parents to be ambivalent toward
their children. But my parents had five kids, and I was by far
the problem child. I was the easy target of their frustration.

My mom would much later reveal that she wished she had
gotten my hormone levels checked, if only she had known
about that sort of thing in those days. She was right.
Something was off in my brain, chemically. Years later I
would be diagnosed with clinical anxiety and depression. But
we didn't know. Assuming I was just a flawed human like the
Bible said, I just learned to live with it.

I am nine, and I am crying. It's my birthday. My mom has
gathered me, my siblings, my cousins, and a friend from
church to go bumper bowling. We arrive at the lanes only to
find out that they lack actual bumpers. Everyone else seems to
bowl better than me. I keep throwing my ball in the gutter.
My mom tries to give me a pointer, which only makes me feel
more like I'm not good enough for her. I sulk off to go buy
licorice. To this day, I still hate bowling. And I still love
licorice.

I am eleven, and I am rehearsing for an upcoming martial arts competition. For hours in my bedroom, I practice the *kata*. I am exhausted, pushing myself to try again and again, until I can perform the entire routine of kicks, punches, and blocks from memory, flawlessly, five times in a row. When the performance arrives, I take first place, beating even my friend April, who is two years older than me. When April's dad picks us up that night, I proudly display my gold medal. Inspecting it, April points out that it isn't made of gold at all, it is made of plastic. "Well, but it's a special kind of plastic," April's dad counters — *Special plastic on a string*. I still feel like a loser.

I am in sixth grade, in my pink-walled bedroom. I am bent over a thin booklet, barely forty pages. It is the Gospel of Luke, from the New Testament. These are the pages I will be quizzed on. I'm holding the book, but my eyes are closed. I'm reciting it from memory, line by line, verse by verse. This is the first year I am officially old enough to compete on the Bible Quiz Team. My goal is to become Rookie of the Year.

In middle school, I am not allowed to post pictures of Hanson or other teenybopper stars in my bedroom, like my friends have done. So I hang every certificate and award I have ever received, a horizontal band of glory wrapped around my bedroom. I display trophies and medals on my dresser. But they aren't enough. I am not enough.

At the age of fourteen, I take the ACT college entrance exam. My score is average. Not good-- average. It shatters my dream of going to the Air Force Academy; I know I need at least a 27 to be considered. I have only scored a 23. I return home that afternoon absolutely crushed. One by one, I remove each certificate of achievement that wraps my bedroom walls, crumpling and throwing away every last one. I crack my journal and solemnly pen yet another melancholy poem:

Papers on the wall
Special plastic on a string
Four long points
Short of my dream

I am 18--how could my fucked up parents still be so
controlling? They hate my boyfriend, and my boyfriend hates
them. No matter what I do, I can't make everyone happy. The
pain cuts through me from the inside out. The pain rages for
expression, but I don't know how to oblige it. My pain won't
act out. I am too well behaved for that. My pain doesn't know
how to scream at my parents or rebel against them. All I know
is that this process hurts, worse than anything I had ever
experienced, and that the pain requires release.

I dig in a drawer for a safety pin. Tears blur my vision. My
hands shake from emotion. The tears don't adequately express
the depth of the pain I feel. So, I seek an instrument of
expression which can fully display my inner turmoil.

My shaking hands pluck a large safety pin from the bathroom
drawer. I retreat to my bedroom and lock the door. Shoving
aside a pile of dirty clothing, I creep to the back of my closet
and shut the bifold doors. In the pitch black, I open the pin
and bend it back. I press the sharp point against my skin. I feel
a pop as the tip punctured the outer layer of the epidermis.
There! There is the expression of the pain. More, there is more.
I drag the pin across my arm slowly. Tracing my finger over
the lines the pin has just drawn on my arm, I feel around in
the darkness for the proof of my pain. And I find it, hot and
wet against my finger.

A few more passes with the pin, and blood stains my jeans.
Deep enough, I have created the experience I was craving. The
shaking leaves my body. A deep breath brings calm. Like a

---

spent lover, I collapse. Emotionless, I am finally able to relax. I pass out with my face in my dirty socks. Maybe now my parents and God and everyone will stop trying to convince me of how much of a loser I am, clearly I already know. It is written all over my arms.

Chapter 2: Gender Identity

"Let a woman learn quietly with all submissiveness. I do not permit a woman to teach or to exercise authority over a man; rather, she is to remain quiet."
1 Timothy 2:11-12

Women have to be nice, quiet, and supportive. A good Christian girl must not ask for anything and must always take less than she really wants, keeping greed in check, especially in a household of seven, don't you dare ask for anything more than your basic needs. Neither should you speak what you mean because you might not sound "nice." Instead, you must read between the lines, speak around the subject, and glean the real truth only from tacit signals. You must never, ever inconvenience someone by wanting something for yourself. Nor should you ever offend someone or inconvenience someone by saying what you mean.

Women should never be idle. They should busy themselves by taking care of others in all moments. Women should not want anything for themselves but always put the needs of others in front of their own. If a woman has a spare moment, she should immediately jump into action, accomplishing something that will benefit others. After all, "Female sluggards chew the cud of gossip and spew the venom of slander" (1 Timothy 5:13).

These ideas were never stated outright. But they didn't need to be. Women were not allowed to be in positions of leadership in my church. The Bible told us that women were to submit to their husbands, that women were created to be the helpers of men. Girls were to remain in the home, under the protection of their fathers, until they were married. My mother reminded me of that when, as a girl, I dreamt out loud about one day having my own apartment. Once married, women were to live under the protection of their husbands. But I think these rules were more about control than protection. Or maybe they were all so scared of my voice that the men used the rules to protect *themselves* from *me*?

Women stood behind men, women supported men, and women were number two. In fact, women were the property of men, a commodity whose value lay in reproduction, cooking, and cleaning. Should we start to value ourselves as anything more than such, we would become very dangerous.

Even at a young age, everything within me hated these ideas. My drive for excellence seemed doomed from the start by my two X chromosomes. As a result, I hated my femininity and rebelled against it at every turn. I arm-wrestled boys in Sunday school and played tackle football with them after church. I followed my older brother and his friends over snowboard jumps in the winter and around the skate park in the summer. The only way I could prove to myself and to the world that I was as valuable as a boy was to compete with them and hold my own. My athletic abilities improved, and any interest in little-girl things never took root.

My mom taught these principles of womanhood and claimed to live by them. But my mom is also highly intelligent and ambitious, which was problematic. Her inner conflict was obvious. She could have risen to become the CEO of a megacorporation or been elected as a high-powered politician. She is that intelligent. My dad, intelligent in a different way, is wise in human relationships. He is sweet, meek, and generous. And he struggled to make C's in college. As a result, my mother passive-aggressively ruled over my dad. I hated seeing this dynamic. Clearly, she was academically smarter than him, and she took every opportunity to show it. Not wanting to provoke her, my dad lived by the motto, "Happy Wife, Happy Life." I remember numerous occasions at the dinner table, jumping to his defense when I could no longer tolerate the way she picked on him.

Freud postulated that gender identity is formed when a child desires the love of their opposite- gendered parent. He said girls desire the love of their fathers. A little girl observes her father's love for her mother. So the girl assumes the characteristics of the mother in order to win her father's love.

I did indeed love my father. And I craved his affection. But I couldn't stand the way Mom treated him. Obviously, a part of her didn't believe she should have to submit to someone she considered beneath her. Religion had robbed my mother of her power. So, she robbed my father of his own power with her incessant belittling. The last thing I wanted was to be like my mother. Of course, I didn't want to be like her; *she* didn't want to be like her. This situation made for a very confusing gender identity.

There were no other females I wanted to be like. I resented my sister for her favored-child status. All the women at the homeschool co-op and church were just like my mom, resentful of what they were forced to become. Most of them carried their resentment in the form of a lot of extra weight. I knew I wasn't going to live that life. But I couldn't conceive of just how much pain breaking out was going to cause me.

One Sunday morning, at age eleven, I battled my mom as we readied ourselves for church. I was trying desperately to get away with wearing pants. I hated wearing dresses. I felt silly and ugly. I felt like I was wearing a Halloween costume--in May. It was awkward and embarrassing. I might as well have been wearing a big red ribbon that said "2nd Place."

"Natasha Marie, you will not wear pants to church!" howled my mom as I came halfway down the stairs.

"But I don't have anything else to wear," I whined back.

"Go upstairs and put on the dress you sewed for the 4-H sewing club."

A homemade dress was the only thing that could possibly be more embarrassing than a regular dress.

"MOM!" I felt sick in my stomach, and I tried to hide my tears. Tears are girly. I hated that I cried so much.

"Natasha," she intoned, exhausted, "God made you a girl for a reason!"

My mom thinks I think I am a boy. I wish I were a boy. Then I could join the football team and quit sewing lessons.

I never wanted to be male, but I definitely never wanted to be what I thought a female was, either. Females were weak. Females were dependent. Females were second-class humans. When I talked to myself in my head, I felt like I was talking to a boy. I knew I wasn't going to be like the older girls and grown women I knew. And so I set out to be strong and independent. I set out, ironically, to be exactly as my mother would have been had her religious beliefs not subdued her. As a kid, I practically took this to mean rejecting all things feminine.

On its own, my belief that I was a wretched sinner was sufficient to fuel my desperate search for validation. Being told that I was a second-class human caused further devastating damage to my developing ego. My resentment toward my mom and her mutual resentment toward me completed the destructive work on my psyche. Any self-esteem I might have developed was stamped out before it had a chance to develop. By the age of twelve, I was desperate for someone to tell me I was lovable. I knew that validation would not come from my parents. And, since men were more valuable than women, the best kind of validation would come from a male.

I assumed that the best way to win the favor of boys was to act like them. After all, why would they be interested in a second-class human? I became very athletic. I suppressed any behavior that could be perceived as needy, emotional, or feminine. Having needs and asking for help was weak. I wanted nothing to do with that. I resolved to be strong and independent. Snowboarding became my outlet. I fell in love with it. When I was on the mountain, dressed in baggy outer gear and a beanie hat, I felt like I fit in. Happily-ever-after was framed for me as a nice husband and a few kids, but I felt like a sinner for having a different vision for my life. My dream was to travel the world as a snowboard bum. I would live in Europe, have a pet monkey, learn to surf in some tropical oasis, and climb the world's highest mountains. I wanted adventure, to taste and see the entire world. Children and marriage were the last things I wanted. My mom did not condone these dreams. There were a series of boxes Christian girls were supposed to check in order to live a happy life. Adventure was not one of them. The relationship between my mother and I devolved into a constant battleground.

As a teen I kept my hair short, I wore baggy clothes, I hated makeup and nail polish, I played guitar in a punk rock band. My mom saw all this as rebellion, which it was: a healthy rebellion against a system that I didn't choose, and that didn't fit me. But I was made to feel like a sinner, which only served to further isolate me. I felt weird and unlovable.

The instant any attention from a boy came my way, I leaped
for it.

Chapter 3: Food, Love, and Mental Illness

"Compulsive eating is only the symptom; believing that you are not worthy of your own love is the problem."
— Geneen Roth

Hospitality is my mom's greatest gift. It's what I admire most in her. She owns and abides in the kitchen. When I was a teenager, my brothers and I would frequently show up at the house with an invasion of hungry friends. Within 10 minutes, a counter full of snacks appeared. My mom makes you chicken salad sandwiches if you are taking a flight. She makes you the world's best enchiladas if you are having surgery. For a funeral, she makes ham sandwiches for hundreds of people. For Thanksgiving, she feeds her entire church, more than 300 people, with turkey and ham and stuffing and mashed potatoes and all the fixings. She graced our backyard sledding parties with warm cookies and hot cocoa. Our summer pool parties received cookies with fresh lemonade. We had family dinner seven days a week, with a meat, a starch, a veggie, and often dessert. Her Sunday dinners are some of my best childhood memories and something still I look forward to when I visit home. She insists on a crisp tablecloth, fine china, crystal glasses, and beautiful serving bowls filled with mashed potatoes, fresh sweet corn, yams, green beans, roast beef, homemade yeast rolls, and jellies she made herself from berries she grew in her own garden. After dinner, my entire family would succumb to a food coma. Scattered around the living room, we'd recline behind glazed eyes, half-watching football, browsing the Sunday paper, half high as a kite.

My mom does not deign to touch, nor does she pay compliments. By contrast, I am a touchy person. I'm a hugger and a cryer. I issue a compliment the minute it hits my brain. Nothing makes me feel loved as much as a hand on my shoulder and a whispered kindness. I can count on one hand the number of times I've heard my mom say I love you. And I've *never* seen her cry. But she does cook, really, really well. And I was starving.

But polite little Christian girls don't ask for favors that might inconvenience someone else. The ultimate value Christianity taught me was that of self-sacrifice. Jesus Christ gave his body as a sacrifice for our sins. I wore a rubber bracelet emblazoned with the letters "WWJD", which stood for What Would Jesus Do? Jesus would be self-sacrificing. This reasoning was invoked when pushing the body to the brink of exhaustion. It was noble to ignore your own desire in service of the greater good.

Mom perfectly modeled this philosophy in her selfless service to the family and the church. Constantly tired she nevertheless endlessly toiled in some way for someone else. She always ate the burnt sandwich or skipped a second helping so there would be more to go around for the rest of us. She never canceled homeschool lessons, even when she was sick. She never took time for herself to exercise or to spend time with friends; others before self always, even if it hurts. After all, the desires of the flesh are evil and cannot be trusted.
The first feeling of "fat" came at the age of 13, when I started to grow into my woman's body. Like most middle school girls, I did carry a little extra plumpness. In the course of three years, my hips, thighs, and butt swelled from a size 0 to a size 11. But my chest didn't keep pace, growing from flat only to a 32 AA, which is to say: I started wearing a bra only because my friends were wearing them, not because there was anything to hold up. This was in the mid-1990s, when slender legs, a vanishing butt, and huge boobs were preferred by men and media. With massive thighs and no boobs at all, my body escaped the attention of the boys.

In a time before hashtags and personally curated social media feeds, my female role models were limited. A few of my friend's moms had jobs outside of the home, but my mother criticized such women. Women were supposed to be moms, not careerists, and moms were supposed to stay home with their kids.

Brief, intermittently allowed glimpses of television or magazines provided my only other examples of adult women. The nineties were not known as a particularly strong time for showcasing women of all sizes, or women in powerful jobs, or even female athletes. My understanding of a woman was either as a repressed, overweight, homeschool moms or the waiflike women who sashayed through pop culture.

I knew I didn't want to be like the subdued, stay-at-home moms I was familiar with. That left either men or wafer-thin supermodels as exemplars. But I was neither male nor thin. I would stew in twenty years of self-hatred before figuring out that all bodies are different, and that such difference is fine. Or more, that I was gifted with an athletic body, strong legs, and a muscular butt deserving of pride.

Hunger presented itself as an enemy shortly after puberty. It would shadow me, constantly tapping on my shoulder. There was never enough, never enough attention, praise, affection, achievements, awards, recognition, or food. I was, after all, a sinner, blemished from birth, a wretch in the eyes of God. I assumed I was hungry because I hadn't earned the right to be recognized or fed. So I worked harder, earned more A's and MVP's. But nothing filled me up.

I won my first battle with hunger when I was 17. After my wisdom teeth were removed, I couldn't eat for a few days. If you've ever fasted or starved yourself, you know that after a day or two it gets a lot easier. And so it did for me. For two days, I couldn't eat due to the pain. But for the two weeks that followed, I didn't eat due to self-hatred.

It felt like a victory. Over the next ten years, I repeated these two-week starvation episodes several times, typically hiding them, even from myself, by calling them "cleanses". But it never seemed to matter whether I gained or lost 10 pounds; I still wasn't full.

Hunger was just another evil impulse from the flesh. It is just an evil impulse from the body that should be ignored or, better yet, punished. I was taught that my body was soiled. Life on earth was putrid and sinful to enjoy, but heaven waited for my soul. I was taught not to become attached to my body or the earth, for they were not my home. The earth will burn, as will the body. The earth and the body are to be subdued.

Much later, I would learn about something called cognitive distortion. Black-and-white thinking is a type of cognitive distortion wherein one labels things as either entirely "bad" or entirely "good." In my thirties, my therapist pointed out that this was an unhealthy way to think. I was blown away. To me, it was the only way to think.

The biggest internal conflict for me became my desire. If I loved Jesus I was supposed to have only pure desires. But I had naughty ones. And they were strong. Eventually, my hunger for recognition and perfect body morphed into a desire for male attention. And since healthy boundaries were never modeled for me, it was only a matter of time before major heartbreak and even abuse entered my life.

Chapter 4: Slut Shame

"In Evangelical culture, an 'impure' girl or woman isn't just seen as damaged; she's considered dangerous. Imagine growing up in a caste and hearing fables about how dragons destroy villages. Then one day, you wake up and see scales on your arms and legs."
Linda Kay Klein
Pure: Inside the Evangelical Movement That Shamed a Generation of Young Women and How I Broke Free

Women's bodies are the most sinful because they harbor the power to corrupt men. Naturally, a religion invented by men in a culture where men are the ruling class would attempt to scare women into vilifying their own bodies. Listening to the body, enjoying its sensations, connecting to nature, following intuition, these were reasons enough for a woman to be executed for witchcraft in early modern Europe. Femininity was a crime punishable by death, and hundreds of thousands of women were hung for it or burned at the stake. Of course, they were--a woman living in full alignment with her personal power is a formidable foe to a complacent male.

All I knew of sex was that it was wrong, dirty, evil, and the worst thing you could do except murder someone. Sex was from Satan, to be entirely avoided in all forms. These forbidden forms included touching a boy in any way more intimate than a brief side hug. Until you got married, that is. At that point, a magical switch would be flipped and all was permitted, as long as you didn't ever talk about it. As long as you never acted publicly in a way that might imply you liked to take off your clothing, behind closed doors with your husband. I wasn't allowed to go on a date or ride in a car alone with a boy until I was eighteen. Skirts had to be knee-length and shirts had to be crew neck; we didn't want to "cause a brother to stumble," as the Bible warns us, now did we?

My religion, although no longer executing women for their femininity, still decreed that embracing the divine feminine would surely result in consignment to hell. A woman capable of expressing her internal strength reminds men that they've been running from their own power. And that is terrifying.

If women's full potential were to be unleashed, then men would also have to be everything they were created to be. Men would have to wake up, open their eyes, shut off the TV, get off the couch, and stop complaining. Keeping the women quiet is much easier. The best way for men to accomplish this is to vilify the kryptonite that threatens them. Obviously, women's sexuality must be repressed. I came to understand that my role was to serve a man; that I must submit my sexual power to the dominant male in my life. That is where my value would be found, in the eyes of a man who found me valuable.

And that is exactly why women who even timidly acknowledged their sex freedom, deserved hell. And why sex was forbidden as the ultimate sin. A woman who wanted anything for herself came in a close second.

When I saw blood in my underwear, I wanted to vomit. I knew what it meant to "pop your cherry," and I swear I hadn't meant to do it. But I let it happen. So it was my fault.

The chain of sin that ended in blood began when I crept from the house under the cover of night. I slid into the tan leather interior of Sam's dad's Lexus. I shook with excitement as Sam planted on me my very first kiss. Sweet sixteen, and never been kissed, up until that moment. But I stiffened when Sam reached up my shirt; I wasn't sure about that part. His breathing descended into a growl. The cute boy I was crushing on transformed into an animal. He started fumbling with my zipper, and I wanted to shout at him to stop. But the good, submissive, quiet little girl couldn't find her words, even as he pushed his hand down the front of my jeans. I was terrified to anger him. Not because I feared he might hurt me, but because I didn't want him to think I wasn't nice. I didn't want him to get mad at me. I didn't want to risk not being liked.

My face contorted into a pucker at the unskilled pawing of his teenaged hands. My stomach clenched in pain when he thrust his middle finger through my innocence. Finally, a fake giggle emerged from me, and I spoke as nicely as I could.

"Sam, slow down."

He looked at me quizzically, then retracted his hand. He said something about how he had to go home, and he kicked me out of the car. Watching him back away, I begged him not to leave. He was mad at me. I had screwed everything up! I returned to my house as furtively as I had exited, through the bathroom window. Bewildered at what had just happened, sick to my stomach for letting it happen, I pulled down my pants to sit on the toilet. That's when I saw the blood. Tears erupted as if to wash away the proof of my sin.

That night would haunt me for years. Each time the youth pastor held forth about staying pure until marriage, I knew I had already gone too far. I confessed to my female youth leader that I had let a guy "go up my shirt." There was no way I could tell her that I had let him finger bang me as well. I said I wanted to become a "second virgin" and asked if she could help me find God's forgiveness. We prayed together. But my repentance did nothing to diminish the weight of the guilt.

Until a month before my eighteenth birthday, I met a guy in a band at a show where I worked backstage, in the hospitality room. He casually asked my age. I said I was eighteen--my birthday was only three weeks away. He was thirty-four. He asked if I wanted to learn some of his band's songs on the guitar. Of course, I did. I also wanted the attention of an older man, a local celebrity. He guided me to a private room and slid a guitar into my hands. Two minutes later, he knocked it out of my hands when he pressed his body over mine. As his hand found the wet folds of my pussy, I awkwardly blurted out the truth in order to escape the situation.

"I'm only seventeen!"

It worked. I fled with my virginity intact, but covered in a new layer of deepest guilt.

That fall, I pressed my face against the floor of a sports stadium packed with 60,000 teenagers. These kids had converged from across the world to attend the "Acquire the Fire" conference. We all wept in unison over our lost innocence. The speaker called to attention anyone who hadn't followed God's commands on sexual purity. Each of the guilty stood, confessing their sin in front of God and everyone. The speaker promised us that, if we confessed publicly, God would forgive us. He said that God would make us pure once more. We could become "second virgins." Ninety percent of the teens in the stadium stood in answer to the call. Although I had never had sex, I had defiled myself, and I wanted to be a virgin again. The speaker commanded us to kneel, to get close to the ground, to make ourselves humble before God. I remember seeing a piece of red hard candy stuck to the floor of the aisle, beside my face. I felt so dirty. I knew I deserved all of this and more.

Many of my friends bought rings from vendors at the conference. Each ring was inscribed with the maxim "True Love Waits." It was to be worn on the left ring finger to symbolize commitment to God. My parents had already purchased me a red ruby "purity ring," which I was already wearing as I pressed my face into the filthy floor.

There were about 50 families involved in my homeschool co-op, and we evolved into a sort of pseudo-school. We had sports teams which played other private schools, and a student council. We had a yearbook and a debate team. The purpose of the debate team was to teach young people how to defend their faith. We spent hours learning logic and reasoning and picking apart each other's arguments. One day, we would become the next generation of great leaders, ready to take back the nation for Christ. So we were taught, and so we believed. The problem with teaching highly intelligent young people to ask questions is that they do just that: ask questions. Questions and faith are intemperate bedfellows.

Throughout high school, my questions grew larger and more existential. One day, I met a gay teenager. And he was cool. He may have been the first authentic human I had ever encountered, living without a mask, without trying to modify who he was in order to gain acceptance. I guess once you've admitted to everyone you like to play with dicks every other aspect of your unique personality is easier to express. I immediately liked him. Why should he go to hell? I had a friend who thought the war in Iraq (which started my junior year) was wrong, and some of his arguments made sense to me. My Catholic grandfather passed away. I hated to think that he might be engulfed in flames because he believed differently and drank beer. Something was missing. Someone wasn't telling me the whole story. Deep in my belly, I felt empty. But I had faith, and that was supposed to fill me up. Surely, something was wrong with me. The quest to find something with which to fill myself persisted.

Obviously, my newfound practice of thinking for myself
didn't go over well with my parents. They hadn't thought for
themselves, ever, and I was a threat. Unfortunately, my
having dismissed everything they taught me about religion
converted them into liars in my eyes. I no longer believed that
they had my best interests at heart. I was smart, too smart. I
pushed them to see what they were missing, and they pushed
harder to control me. They held money over me. My car, my
college tuition, gas money...I would get none of it if I didn't do
exactly as I was told.

While in college, I began to attend a new church. The church
was called Mars Hill and was led by a guy named Rob Bell.
Rob sounded different from anyone I had ever heard in a
church. He talked about how the Bible was a collection of
ancient poems and letters and was never meant to be a
textbook or instruction manual. He taught one particularly
provocative series on the role of women in the church. He
used the Bible in a new way---to argue for gender equality. He
also taught a series called "God is Green", arguing for
protecting the environment. This argument stood in contrast
to the "it's all going to burn" message I had previously heard
in church. Groups of protesters started to form outside the
church doors. We had to walk through them in order to
return to our cars after services. Rob taught things none of us
had ever heard from the pulpit. His lessons went against
everything I had ever been taught. And, in my bones, they felt
right.

This was the first time I heard the idea that it was okay to be
female and okay to embrace physical form as sacred. My mom
would always say, "If it's not from God, then where is it from?
The devil." The idea that the environment was sacred was

earth-shaking. Could my body be sacred too? It would be years before these ideas would really sink in, but the seeds had been planted.

I felt either that I was broken and couldn't make the system work, or that the system itself was broken. Starting to explore outside the lines of mainstream Christianity, I read fringe Christian authors, each one challenging me to think a little bigger. I hid these books from my mother. I credit Rob Bell and Brian McLaren for my status as a "Recovering Evangelical." I discovered that I wasn't the only one with the icky gut feeling that I wasn't being told the whole story, and this revelation gave me immense comfort. But, once I accepted that there was more to the story, I experienced an awful sensation of my entire foundation crumbling. Christianity was all or nothing. You had to accept it on faith and not allow yourself to question it. But the story had too many holes in it to hold water. I felt like I was sinking.

During my senior year of high school, one of my best friends, Merideth, who was naturally gorgeous and sexy, got into stripping. She had a rough home life and had been emancipated at 17. Dancing was an easy way for her to earn her own money. I was shocked, appalled, and secretly jealous. I thought about how much fun she must be having, turning on all those guys, and getting paid for it. But I never admitted to those thoughts, not even to myself. I never gave them words. They never emerged in a private journal entry. But I definitely had them. I wished I could do what Merideth did. But, of course, I never seriously considered that I could strip if I wanted to. Wishing to be a dancer was like wishing to be Angelina Jolie; I'd need to have been born a completely different person. In reality, all I had to do was go down to the local titty bar and audition. That thought never once entered my head. It was just off-limits.

After high school, I went on to study math and physics, the most masculine major I could find. Maybe then I would be enough? I got a job in my home town, making $32,000 annually. Merideth moved to Pennsylvania and became one of the most popular entertainers in Philly. Her lingerie-clad body stretched along the sides of buses. I always respected her bravery in posting all of her exploits on her public Facebook. Merideth didn't give a shit. In fact, Merideth loved it. She owned every inch of herself, inside and out. In doing so, she became far sexier than I was able to be.

Even at the time, I knew I was jealous. Part of me was jealous because she was so sexy, far sexier than I was. But even more, I was jealous because she was doing something I wanted to do, but had no way of admitting to myself that I wanted to do it. I wanted to be sexy. I wanted lots of money. I wanted to see the world. I wanted guys to want me so badly that they would pay good money to have me rub up on them. That would make me valuable. I wanted her gall. But I repressed my desires so much that I never even considered it an option. Instead, I studied hard, got good grades, and tried my best to stay thin so I could find a good husband.

Chapter 5: Diet Culture

Diet culture is a system of beliefs that worships thinness and equates it to health and moral virtue, which means you can spend your whole life thinking you're irreparably broken just because you don't look like the impossibly thin "ideal." -Christy Harrison, Intuitive Eating

My mom, like most of the corn-fed midwestern women in her church, was neither thin nor happy. These subdued, asexual people were not the pattern of femininity that I wanted to follow. That much was clear. I swore I would be nothing like them, no matter how much it cost me.

Watching your weight was an acceptable part of the culture around me. It seemed perfectly normal to be unhappy with your weight unless you looked like a fashion model. I therefore assumed there was an ideal size to be, just as Jesus was the model of the ideal person, A's were the ideals of a good student, MVP was the ideal of an athlete and fashion models were the idea of perfect bodies. Anything less than the ideal was wrong, and it was my own fault. But I was athletic. My calf muscles didn't fit into the flared-leg jeans that were popular when I was a teenager. My biceps didn't fit into the sleeves on my formal gown. It never occurred to me that my body type was different from that of a fashion model. Or if it did, I assumed it was because I had done something wrong. I must have eaten too much. The instant I grew hips, I began to hate my body.

I was around 16 when I started to exert willpower over my hunger. I was accustomed to mind-over-mattering my way toward getting the job done. I was well versed in the virtue of denying the needs of the body. After all, bodies were the entry point for danger. It was much safer to just control them. Being no stranger to discomfort for the sake of righteousness, I found it no stretch at all to label my hunger as bad, especially when dieting pervaded the culture around me.

Mindy, a delicate, non-athletic 15-year-old and the most popular girl at the homeschool co-op, made sure to point out that the muffin I was eating had almost 400 calories. I made sure to eat only half while anyone was watching.

"This is gross," I told the other girls at the table, "Anyone want the rest?" I made a show of not eating the entire muffin. There were no takers. *Now what?* I couldn't bring myself to throw it out, especially not with my stomach still growling. I wrapped the half muffin in a napkin and walked toward the trash. When I reached the trash, I threw away only the napkin and held the rest of the muffin out of the sight of Mindy and the other skinny girls. I carried the remaining muffin with me to the bathroom and, safely hidden behind the stall door, scarfed it down. I made sure my feet were pointing forward so that, in case anyone walked in, they wouldn't wonder what I was doing. It felt dirty and wrong and oh so pleasurable.

My first real excursion into eating disorder behavior occurred when I was an undergraduate. I found the willpower to live on Jell-O, cottage cheese, carrot sticks, and coffee for almost 6 weeks. I allowed myself 600 calories per day unless I went for a 3-mile walk while carrying hand weights. In that case, I could have 800 calories. To me, nothing seemed unusual about my behavior. I felt guilty, not because I was starving myself, but because I wasn't thin. My body was so flawed that it kept making me feel hungry when I clearly had weight to lose.

As my extreme diet caused some of my natural muscle to wither, for the first time in my life, the scale started to drop. I felt victorious. I continued to ignore my hunger for the

remainder of my college years. I began to exercise
compulsively. I trained for and ran marathons to help keep
the weight off. Running for hours a day, giving up weekends
to do long runs, never staying out late with friends...it all
seemed like a small price to pay for beauty.

One college roommate showed me how to use soup broth as a
meal replacement. One bouillon cube and hot water, and you
had dinner with less than 10 calories! She was incredibly thin
and constantly had boys over to our dorm. She seemed to
really know what she was doing. Another roommate replaced
her meals with coffee or alcohol. Nothing I was doing seemed
out of the ordinary. Most of my friends were also "eating
clean" or "cutting back", as we called it. Diet culture was all
we knew. But we never called it "dieting"; that was what our
mothers did. We knew better than to go on a *diet*. We were
"living a healthy lifestyle." If you were hungry, it was easy to
label the hunger as just another "urge" arising from your bad
body. Being hungry didn't mean you needed to eat. Eating
meant caving into the flesh.

For me, being thin was always about getting male attention. If
men desired me, then I was valuable. Then I had duped the
system. Though religion attempted to maintain male power
by erasing my sexual power, I still recognized what my
sexuality could accomplish. But it wasn't just religious culture
that feared a woman's sexuality. Misogyny was a part of the
culture as a whole. The best way to keep a woman from using
her sexual power is to make it seem immoral. Beauty is
reserved for only the most perfect of females. Only the
helpless, tiny, waif-like, unintelligent women get to wear the
badge of attractiveness. And I bought it. The best way to be a
worthwhile female was to be small.

There was some kind of security to be found in beauty. If I
was thin and therefore beautiful, then I could choose who I

would marry. I would not have to settle. I could be with a rich man, a successful man. My life would be complete. I would have followed the prescribed path and happily-ever-after would be mine. Everything hinged on getting boys to like me. But who would like me unless I was first thin?

Chapter 6: Consent

"We have English 101 together, right?"

He questioned from his seat beside me on the park bench.
"You always sit in the front and answer all the questions.
What, are you some kinda genius? You look like you're 14."

"I'm 16, and I'm homeschooled. So my parents just enrolled
me in community college rather than having me finish out
high school."

"Oh, well, I like your skirt. You ever wear it without
underwear?"

"What? Um, no, I guess not."

"Will you? Tomorrow, come to class in a skirt and no panties.
That'd be hot!"

"Um, I don't know." I looked down at my lunch. I liked the
attention, but it felt creepy at the same time.

"Nice banana. I like how you are eating it." He kept on.

"That's just how you eat bananas. I mean, you just peel them
and take a bite. Everyone eats bananas like that." He was
embarrassing me, but it didn't occur to me simply to get up
and walk away. Or better yet, tell him to fuck off. I didn't
want to offend him.

"Yeah, you should take a really big bite. Like, see how much
you can get in your mouth at once."
It felt like he was making a sexual comment and I felt violated.
But I wasn't sure if this was just some public school joke I had

missed out on and would then look very silly if I didn't play along.

But that was the last time I brought a banana to school. The attention did feel good. That guy started to sit next to me in class. He convinced me to sit in the back row with him. It wasn't hard, he just told me to. I didn't know how to say no. He kept telling me to wear no panties. I didn't want to, but he insisted. I didn't have any other friends, and I was afraid the attention would stop if I refused him. So, one day I took off my panties just before class and proudly announced to him that I wasn't wearing anything under my skirt. He dug in his bag as I took my seat next to him. A few minutes into class, I noticed him stretching his feet out in front of him. Tucked into his shoelaces was a tiny mirror. I crossed my legs.

—

Jackson was my first real boyfriend. The event marked my eighteenth year. None of my friends liked him. My parents hated him. I'm not sure even I liked him. But he liked me. And I had never experienced a boy pursuing me. Jackson drank heavily, smoked cigarettes, and dropped out of high school his senior year. But he also led worship at a church and was the son of a pastor. Seeing him on a stage, playing guitar, and singing praise to Jesus, got me all sorts of worked up. My sister had married a worship leader and my parents couldn't have been more proud of her. At the time, I was just beginning to explore my femininity. Jackson found me attractive when many others did not. The attention was addictive.

We met when he was a guest worship leader at my parents' church, where I played bass guitar every other Sunday morning. We went on to lead worship together at churches all over the city. We talked about taking adventures together, road-tripping to California, or becoming ski bums in Canada.

Suddenly, the idea of marriage and its promise of happily ever after weren't in conflict with my heart's desire for adventure. I could see that a way might exist for me to have both what I wanted and what my parents told me I should I want.

One night after rehearsal, when the rest of the praise team had gone, we climbed into the back seat of his car and started steaming up the windows. Things got hotter and steamier, and through my jeans something crazy happened. Something inside me felt like an explosion, and shook my body in the best kind of way. I had no idea what was happening to me. Then, as soon as it started, it stopped. Euphoria was instantly replaced with a sickening guilt in the pit of my stomach, so deep it would haunt me for years.

Jackson kept trying to do more and more with me each time we steamed up the car. I was never taught how to say no when someone wanted something from me, Christians don't do a lot of no-saying. Of course, I wanted it too. But my desire was overshadowed by the guilt which controlled my life. So, although I told Jackson no, I said it through laughter, terrified he might not like me anymore if I really held my ground. Of course, he ignored my weak-throated protests and proceeded to take what he wanted. Afterward, I would insist it could never happen again. But again and again, it would happen, each time a little more. Each time, the guilt would make me physically ill. My stomach would tighten into knots, acid churning, burning my innards. Only starchy foods seemed to help neutralize the acid. Jackson would drop me off for my 11:00 PM curfew, and I would go straight to the kitchen, nauseous and starving. I'd wake up in the morning with that same sickening feeling. Nearly every hour, a wave of guilt would grip my innards and I'd go looking for a snack. This guilt-driven appetite would persist for the next ten years.

One day, I came home to a quiet house after class at community college. I phoned my mom to inquire where everyone was. She informed me she was in the hospital with my 15-year-old brother. He was in the ICU with bacterial meningitis. He was in critical condition. It was serious. My mom sounded shaken up. My mom doesn't get shaken up. I called Jackson for some emotional support and he rushed to my parents' house. Terrified for my brother, I cried in his arms.

"You know what will make you feel better?" he said, "if we get naked." I told him that was not what I wanted. That it would not make me feel better, but worse. He pushed and he pushed. Overwhelmed by what was going on, just trying not to upset him, I found it easier to stop arguing and just get it over with. That day I lost both my virginity and my freedom. Guilt became my prison.

One freezing winter night, we got into a fight (yet another) about who-knows-what. Sitting in the car with the heater running, he launched into another of his head games.

"If you really were committed to me, then you would marry me."

"I will marry you, but what's the rush?" I was 18, he was 17.

"Then we can get a place together and we won't have to deal with your insane parents and sneaking around. Marry me. Marry me tomorrow. Marry me tomorrow or leave me tonight, up to you."

At 17, he was a minor and would need the signature of his parents. So, at 11:00 PM, we drove to his house, got his parents out of bed, announced we were getting married in the morning, and requested a permission slip. Jackson's dad agreed on one condition: we had to tell my parents as well.

My mom tightened her robe. My dad folded his arms across his big chest. They sat across from us at the dining room table, completely annoyed at being awakened at midnight on a Tuesday. What happened next is a bit of a blur. I remember Jackson telling my dad that he was marrying me in the morning. My dad told him that was absolutely not going to happen. An argument followed and we stood up to go. My mom lunged at me as we made our way to the door. She tackled me, and we wound up in a heap on the floor. I didn't fight back. I was bigger than my mom and I didn't want to hurt her, nor did I really want to win the fight. The last time my mom held me in her arms, I was a toddler. At that moment, I was fine right there in her grip on the dining room floor. My dad, at 6 foot 2 and 215 pounds, picked up Jackson like the little shit he was and flung him out the front door. But Jackson wasn't giving up. He drew back his fist and reminded my dad that he was only a minor, so my dad better not hurt him. He then proceeded to clock my dad in the eye. Somehow, Jackson and I ended up out the door, driving a short distance to safety, where he parked the car. I cried until I hyperventilated and passed out.

We did not end up getting married that morning. My parents made me an offer I could not refuse. In order to get me away from my boyfriend, they offered to send me to a college out of state. Any college, as long as it was Christian. My heart's desire was a snowy mountain adventure away from my hometown, off on my own. My parents were offering to make it happen. I chose a school outside of Denver, where I could snowboard four days per week. My semester there should have been a dream come true, but instead, I spent three hours every night on the phone with my boyfriend. I never made any new friends. Overwhelmed by loneliness, I returned to be near Jackson after one semester.

A year later, I was still trying to break it off with him. My perfect, oldest sister was pregnant with her first child. She had married her high school sweetheart, having saved herself for her husband, even after ten years of dating. They bought a house, and everyone was eagerly anticipating the family's first grandbaby. She was living the textbook happily-ever-after scenario. On the day the baby was to be born, my parents went to the hospital for the birth. I went to find Jackson, who hadn't returned my previous night's phone calls. I found his apartment strewn with liquor bottles and women's clothing. I walked into his bedroom. He lay on a bare mattress on the floor, passed out with a naked girl next to him. "Wow," is all I said. Just like that, it was over.

In the face of what I had just seen, news of my sister's labor was too much for my teenage soul to bear. I was ruined. I had been justifying my premarital sex to myself by insisting that we were married in God's eyes; soon enough, we would be married in the eyes of the state as well. The Bible teaches that if a woman gets a divorce, she should remain single. To do otherwise is adultery. So that was that. I was no longer going to be with Jackson and I could never be with another man. I was never going to get married. I would never, like my perfect sister was doing, give my parents a grandchild. I had committed an unforgivable sin. My life was over. Why bother living another day?

I found a big container of over-the-counter pills in my parents' medicine cabinet. I knew the Bible said that "If we confess our sins...He will cleanse us from all unrighteousness." But how could I confess to what I had done? Confessing to God was one thing, but somehow I felt the only way to be forgiven was to confess to my mother. I would rather die.

Every five minutes, I swallowed another pill. I was putting my life in the hands of time: either my mom would come home and find me and I would confess...or I would die before she returned.

I knew about what time she would be home. I made sure I didn't have enough time to do any real damage. I was about 8 or 9 pills in when I heard the garage door open. I made a display of my remorse with the open bottle of pills and the half-empty glass of water.

I wept and she held me. She felt warm.

I said I hated myself and I wanted to die. She said she loved me.

"I had sex, Mom."

"I know, God can forgive you," she said, and she held me tighter.

Chapter 7: Toxic Christian Guilt

"Just because someone isn't willing or able to love us, it doesn't mean that we are unlovable." Brené Brown

Josh called me "woman" and grunted at me when he wanted something from me. And I liked it. I married Josh when I was most desperate for male validation. And Sex. Josh and I started sleeping together the summer before my senior year of college. We never really dated; we just went to basement drinking parties and then fucked. Josh was just about as desperate for female attention as I was for male attention. He had been the classic, glasses-wearing, bookworm, dork in his small Christian high school. He began drinking heavily to try to fit in. He lost his driver's license due to DUIs in college. He was now a college dropout bumming rides off his little brothers to work in the family manufacturing factory. Each of our neediness fed the other.

Eventually, Christian guilt over our hooking up overwhelmed us both. He proposed and I accepted. I hoped that getting back on the straight and narrow path would lead to the happiness and fulfillment I was desperately missing.

My wedding was in two days. Close to four hundred People had RSVPed. Details were arranged, caterers paid, my parents' backyard was perfectly manicured.
And I was crying.

Was it cold feet or was it something more? I had just returned from Josh's house, which in two days would also be my house. He was on his way home from work, so I let myself in with my key and started cooking dinner. I hoped we could discuss some last-minute wedding details. He arrived to the smell of garlic and onion frying in a pan of butter. He was grumpy. He seemed upset that I was there. He didn't say it, but he didn't have to. He wanted his space. I hadn't seen him for two days. It seemed like forever to me, but apparently he didn't feel the same way. He unpacked his computer from his backpack and, pushing aside the plates I had set out for dinner, he set up his video game station at the dinner table. He said he wasn't hungry. I made myself a plate of food and sat next to him. I ate without talking, listening to the sound of his mouse clicks and the slashing of a stupid digital sword as he hacked down some stupid digital monsters. I cleaned the kitchen, put the leftovers in the fridge, and returned in tears to my friend's house, where I was renting a room until the wedding.

Two days later, I stood in front of all my friends and family and promised to love Josh until death do us part. I was beautiful: daisies in my hair and a huge white dress. The wedding was in the woods, by a creek in my parents' backyard. My dad and I descended a rolling green hill behind the guests for my big entrance. We feasted on a pig named Roy that my younger brother had raised for 4-H. All that attention; it was one of the best days of my life.

Josh and I had rushed things, of course. I knew it, my parents knew it, my friends knew it, and Josh knew it. But, once the ring was on my finger, I had no idea how to say no. I didn't want to be married. I wanted adventure, risk, and travel. I wanted to have sex with lots of people, although I could have never admitted it to myself at the time. But marriage was what I was supposed to do. I wanted the happily ever after that marriage promised. I'm sure Josh probably felt the same way. We both had been raised with strict Christian values; neither of us valued ourselves enough to know how to say what we wanted. We did, however, know that we wanted to have sex, and in order to do that without guilt, we would need to get married. So we did.

A couple of months into our marriage, before our move to San Diego, I lay awake in our bed while Josh played video games in the other room. This had become a pattern. I would go to bed alone, wanting sex, while he would stay up late staring at a screen. I was overwhelmingly lonely, waiting in our freezing Michigan home for him to come join me. But I said nothing and waited patiently, like good Christian wives do. Eventually, he pulled back the covers and slid into his side of the bed, his butt facing me. I rolled toward him and attempted to be the big spoon. He shook his body and moved away from me. This was the fifth night in a row my brand new husband would come to bed late, not in the mood for sex. I lay there, just a few inches away from him, feeling more alone than ever before. My body screamed, "Don't you see me! I'm right here waiting for you to want me!" But my voice said nothing. Tension in my chest choked the words from me. In reality, I expected that he would read my mind. He, of course, did not.

I felt him yelling, "You are fat and needy, get off me!" Which, of course, he did not say at all, but it tacitly filled my ears nonetheless. Hot tears stung my eyes, but I was used to it. I couldn't understand how playing video games could possibly be better than coming to bed with your new bride. I was devastated. We were 21 and 27 years old, evangelical Christians who believed sex should be reserved for marriage. We had fought our urges for our entire engagement. Now, not three months into the marriage, the entire reason for it seemed to be gone.

My tears turned to silent sobbing, which I knew he could feel from his side of the bed. He didn't move, even though I could tell from his breathing that he was still awake. The sobbing got worse and the ignoring got louder until I got out of bed and headed for the bathroom.

As I passed the living room, the glaring blue light from Josh's computer hurt my eyes. I walked over to shut the lid, but then remembered he had been in the middle of a game. I didn't want to shut it down in case he was letting it run overnight to gain some kind of points or for some other stupid video game reason. I bumped the mouse to wake up the screen.

My story is all too common. I don't even need to describe what I saw there. It wasn't a video game.

My sheltered little Christian heart dropped to the floor and shattered into a million little pieces. I left my heart on the floor, entered the bathroom, drank half a bottle of cold medication, and pulled a towel over me. I woke up shivering in the daylight. I wanted nothing more than to be dead.

I didn't confront Josh right away the next day, nor did he ask why I had stayed the night in the bathroom. We went about our morning, as usual, screaming at each other from our mutually silent mouths. The next chance I got, I examined his browsing history and clicked on every image he had viewed. I compared myself to each and every one, noticing if my stomach was flatter or if my thighs were smaller. Josh had been lying to me about what he was doing, for months choosing other women on a screen over my body. It felt like betrayal, it felt like adultery, it felt like my fault. If only (as he would later tell me) my butt was smaller and my boobs were bigger, then he would choose me over them.

A few nights later, we were out at a craft brewery with close friends. A woman I didn't know was hanging around our group. She had perfect boobs and a tight little butt. Josh kept calling her "sweety" and "hon". He called all the girls like that. It pissed me off. He kept finding a reason to talk to her. At one point, she made a joke at his expense. She was flirting and he was eating it up. Up until that point I had silently ignored her. When she made a sarcastic comment about my husband, I lost my mind. She was standing, and I stood up to tower over her in my heels. Although I was far from drunk, I knocked the beer out of her hand and began screaming, *screaming*, in a crowded brewery. All the words I had been holding in finally erupted, directed at some poor innocent girl. The simple fact that she was attractive made her my enemy. I don't remember what I said, but it was something about ripping off her perfect tits if she took one step closer. I am a good Christian girl with wholesome parents and conservative values. This outrage from within me scared me more than anyone on the outside could ever do.

The next morning, some friends who had been there that night suggested I get help. I agreed. That was the first of many times that I sought counseling.

For the next two years, I wanted out. He probably did too. I didn't like what I had signed up for. We had some good days, but not many. We moved to California, fulfilling a dream I'd had for years. I had always wanted to be a surfer. But instead of living by the ocean, we lived with roaches in a grubby inner-city apartment. It was all we could afford. I was in grad school and he refused to work more than 15 hours per week. Mostly, it was two years of me working on my graduate studies, ignoring him playing video games, and him ignoring me while I slept alone. Josh tried to blame his lack of sexual interest in me on my appearance. He said my body type just didn't interest him. He was a "boob man" and I was a booty girl. So I also got a third job as a waitress--while still tutoring, teaching undergraduate classes, and taking graduate coursework--to save for a breast augmentation. And I redoubled my unhealthy commitment to exercise.

I started exercising at least twice a day during my grad school years, no matter how exhausted I was. Eventually, Josh and I nearly stopped talking. He played a lot of video games and I spent a lot of time solving math problems, at work and at the gym. For the two years that we were married, I can count on one hand the number of times I had my shirt off during sex. Josh never touched my breasts before my augmentation. I don't ever recall him giving me oral sex. The number of times he asked me for a blow job, however, was multiple per day. Most of the time, I performed oral sex on him and then we were done. If we did have vaginal intercourse it was from behind, spooning, or doggy style. For the most part, I turned off my urges. But sometimes they became too much to handle.

When Josh was at work, I occasionally played around on a video chat website where you were matched up with a random stranger. Obviously, it became a place for video sex. When I couldn't deal with my sexual urges anymore, the idea of that website wouldn't leave my mind until I finally gave in. For free, I would take off my clothing and point the camera toward my pussy; I loved every second of it. To see a man so horny for me that he would masturbate just at the sight of me made me feel as powerful as those pornstars my husband preferred over me. I knew of girls doing this on websites for pay. Of course, I could never do that. I thought it sounded fun, all that attention and easy money. But again, I never allowed myself to own this thought. I pushed it out of my mind the instant it entered.

Josh and I admitted there was a problem with our sex life. I was devastated by him choosing porn over me. I racked my brain trying to find a solution. The part of me that craved sexual adventure was willing to try anything. I believe it was Josh's idea, although it could have been mine, to try a threesome.

This is easier said than done. We hunted around on Craigslist for a while. I even went alone on a very awkward date with a woman to a nude beach. She wanted to meet me first, before agreeing to meet Josh. She was beautiful, to be sure, but I had no sexual desire for her. We spread our towels out on Black's beach in La Jolla. I immediately stripped all the way down and then felt awkward when she took off only her top. I put my bottoms back on. I remember walking up the beach stairs to leave, making some totally contrived comment about how I was getting turned on by watching her butt. It wasn't true, but I knew I had to do something to get her to like me enough to want to meet Josh. It felt gross to hear the untrue words coming out of my mouth. Nothing more ever came of our meeting.

We continued our hunt, now at gay bars, seeking a woman willing to go to bed with us. I was always amazed at how much Josh seemed to enjoy dancing with other men. I couldn't believe how open-minded he was. One night, we did meet a woman who invited us back to her house after we'd all been drinking heavily. She clearly told us that she was lesbian, not bisexual, and would only have sex with me. She said my husband could watch. He agreed. But when we got to her house, she pulled me into her room and closed the door, leaving Josh sitting in the kitchen in the dark. I think she must have gone down on me, although I don't really remember. I definitely remember going down on her. I didn't care for it much. It didn't bother me, but I certainly wasn't into it. I was just doing my duty, same as I did for my husband after the fifth time he asked me for oral sex daily. When I left her room, my husband was missing. I drove home and found the apartment empty. An hour or so later, he showed up. He had walked over four miles. He said he heard me in there "cheating" on him, and he couldn't take any more of it so he left. His comments devastated me. I had just performed a sex act I didn't want to do for the sake of my marriage, and now he was calling it cheating. After that, sex became nearly non-existent between us.

Things were spiraling downward quickly. It was my last semester of graduate school, and my desire for adventure still tapped on my shoulder. And attached to the desire for adventure, a dormant desire for wild sex lay hidden even from myself. I felt stuck in my marriage. I suggested we apply to the Peace Corps. Josh liked this idea, so we applied together and were approved. We were given an assignment in western Africa and were slated to leave the fall following my graduation. At last, my thirst for adventure would be quenched!

But that last semester would prove to be a long one. Around that time, Josh decided that God had commanded him to quit drinking and smoking weed. What I didn't understand at the time was that his substance abuse was actually self-medication for a very serious mental illness. He had always been quite depressed, but when he stopped using, the illness which had been progressing, started to show clearly. One day, he pointed out a white van that had been parked in the neighbor's driveway for a couple of days. He said it was filled with government agents who were looking for him. The next day, I opened my computer to find tape over the webcam. He had done the same to his own computer and both our phones as well. A few days later, I came home to find over 100 sticky notes slapped all over the house with messages like, "God is watching" and "Jesus cares" scrawled all over them. Soon he grew paranoid about me. He was convinced I was sleeping with his best friend. I came home with a scratch on my shoulder, and he used it as evidence against me. I had a tank top that I had cut and tied back together to fit tighter. Josh was sure someone with whom I was sleeping had torn it off of me, and that is why I had to tie it.

Just before Christmas, Josh announced the truth.

"I've been using my external hard drive when I browse porn, so nothing gets traced to the computer. That's why I don't need to erase the browser history. I'm done. I can't be with you. I can never forgive you for cheating on me. I'm going to file for divorce." He stated it simply, without emotion, as if he were telling me what he had for lunch.

The feeling in my body shocked me more than the words he spoke. I didn't feel sad or betrayed. I felt relieved, and a little pissed, but mostly relieved. At last, it was over. And what was better, he was doing the leaving, not me. Neither God nor my parents could fault me for this. There would be no Peace Corps, but finally, I would be free to live whatever adventure I wanted. The problem now was admitting to myself what it was I really wanted.

Calling my mother to tell her I was getting a divorce was perhaps the first truly brave thing I have ever done. They say change only happens when the fear of the unknown is outweighed than the misery of the present. After accepting the shame of divorce, acting upon many things I had always wanted but was too ashamed to try seems comparatively easy. I was one step closer to following my heart, which had been shut off years and years ago.

Chapter 8: Wild Oats

I was ripe to explore my urges for men and for adventure. I was in a new job that required weekly travel. This job came with a bigger paycheck, a sexy new wardrobe, a cute new car, and a classier new apartment. With Josh, I worked hard to improve my appearance in order to draw him toward me. In addition to getting breast implants, I lost and kept off ten pounds, grew my hair out, and learned how to wear nail polish, earrings, makeup, and heels. In my marriage, I had collected brand new sexual experiences and dropped a great deal of the shame surrounding the subject. But the biggest change of all was in my confidence. I had built up enough self-assurance to break the rules I grew up with.

I was ready to slowly explore my sexual freedom. For the first time, casual sex became an option. But, though I was growing bolder, my guilt persisted. I experienced desires but I couldn't own them: I wanted sex; I wanted dirty sex, a lot of it - raw, unbeautiful sex. I wanted to binge on sex. I wanted to have sex with anyone I wanted, whenever I wanted. I was 25, a size 6 with DD's and a pleasing personality. I could have entered any bar, any night of the week and emerge with a sexual partner. But I neither knew that, nor would I have been capable of actually doing it, even though I desperately wanted it. So, within a few weeks, I jumped into a committed relationship with a man who seemed nice enough. He couldn't keep his hands off of me, which addressed my still lacking self-esteem. He rode a Harley and took me on all kinds of adventures, skydiving, jet-skiing the Colorado River, and snowboarding in the local mountains. It was exactly what I craved--except for the monogamy. I am ashamed to confess that I cheated on that boyfriend several times, engaging in one night stands while I traveled for business.

On one particular night, I knew exactly what I wanted. My sexual guilt was vanishingly small and my desire for risky, adventurous sex was peaking. I was staying in a crappy little Arizona town for a work trip. I crossed the street from my hotel to slip into a dive bar, still wearing my work outfit: a pencil skirt and heels. I had abandoned the blazer, and my bare shoulders were exposed. I ordered a vodka soda and surveyed the bar. Locating the most attractive man, I decided that he would be my evening's plaything. He was shooting pool. I ordered two shots of tequila and change for a dollar. I hiked my skirt a little higher, tugged my blouse a little lower, and moved to the pool table. Drink in one hand, four quarters and two shots in the other, I arrived at the rail of the table and set down my cargo. Startled, the attractive man raised his eyes.

"Cheers and I'm playing the winner." I gifted him a flirty smile, pushed one of the shots his way, and threw back my own.

Several more drinks helped drown the guilt I felt about inviting him back to my room. I have no memory of what happened until the next morning. When the alarm went off at 5:00 am, a sickening guilt suffused my body, competing with gut rot and a killer headache for my miserable attention.

The boyfriend I was cheating on convinced me to compete in a beauty contest. I would parade in front of thousands of people, clad in bikini and heels. The winner would become a spokesmodel for the contest organization, making appearances at charity events alongside other bikini-wrapped winners. Hoping my parents would never find out, I entered the contest.

In the evening of the contest, I was in full costume: hair, nails, makeup, heels, tan, jewelry, pasted-on smile. I was called to stage along with the other contestants for some parading around. Then we were dismissed backstage. We waited, breathless, as they called the four finalists back on to the stage. I almost choked when I heard my name. I strutted back out, into the glaring lights, performing a little twirl, certain I was going to puke. I reminded myself that being a finalist was good enough. Just being a finalist meant that I was already prettier than almost everyone else. But I knew in my heart that second place would feel like first place loser. They called the name of the second runner up, then the name of the first runner up. Neither of these names was mine. There were just two of us left. I looked at the other girl whose name had not been called. She was pretty, but I was prettier and I knew it.

Receiving that bouquet of flowers, that crown, that blue satin sash...well, it changed everything. My whole life up until that moment, I had believed I was ugly and I had placed all my energy into validating my existence on earth through other endeavors. Awards and trophies, first places and championships for sports and academics...all of it meant nothing if I was fat and ugly. And now, at last, I was not just a beautiful woman, I was more beautiful than the others. I had been seen.

For a few months, my unhealthy relationship with food and exercise took a backseat. I reveled in the glory of my crown, my sash, and my boyfriend, who worshiped at my feet. A few pounds crept back on as I drank bottomless mimosas and went for Harley rides--instead of trail runs--with my boyfriend. Eventually, I was scheduled for a photo shoot for the organization with which I was a spokesmodel. It was spring. I realized that I had packed on some winter weight. I went searching for the next great diet to get ready for my shoot. What I found would change my life forever.

I read a book by a doctor who claimed that humans do not

need to eat carbohydrates. Further, he claimed that carbs are the cause of fat storage. I had tried everything else. I was desperate for something that worked. So I cut out a lot of junk like taco shops and drive-through food, but I also cut out all whole grains, all fruit, and almost all veggies. I pretty much ate only meat and oil. There was nothing "living" in my diet. Within three days, my hunger had shut down and I lost several pounds.

It was the magic bullet. The more success I tasted, the more driven I became. I started exercising more and more, and I prided myself in exercising on an empty stomach, so the only fuel to burn was stored fat. I started surfing. I would wake up early, walk the beach, and surf. I would work a few hours on my computer, do a Crossfit workout on the beach, work a few more hours, and go for a 3-5 mile run. I was exercising 4-5 hours daily. With a calorie counting app, I tracked every bite of food that went into my mouth. I weighed and measured every portion. I quit eating out and I quit drinking. I was thin enough before I started my no-carb diet, at my natural weight, but I lost another 25 pounds. Once, I Googled "average height and weight of a Victoria's Secret model"... and I had arrived!

That first summer, when I reached my goal weight, was one of the happiest in memory. I broke up with my not-so-hot boyfriend, mostly because for the first time in my life there were so many new options. Looking back, I don't think it was my weight that got me all the additional male attention. Much more, it was a newfound confidence in my body and an uplifted personality. I was thin. Therefore I was good. I was comfortable in my own skin for the first time in 15 years. My attitude--not my overly thin body--oozed sex appeal. I finally had what I wanted. I was getting asked out on dates right and left. Attention came from all sides. Finally, I was a woman in control of her sexual power, except for all the guilt still lingering just beneath the surface. I was still apprehensive to

wield my power. Knowing what greatness you are capable of
and lacking the bravery to follow through is one of the
weakest places a human can live. So I would become the
frailest version of myself.

Chapter 9: Guilted Back into Monogamy

One of my new admirers eyed me from under his flat bill. I
was in my backyard, working simultaneously on my
computer and my tan. He chatted with my neighbor. Each
time I lifted my eyes from the screen, I caught him gazing at
me. His eyes would dart back to the ground. He had that
signature SoCal, surfer, bad-boy look: tattoo sleeves, Dickies
shorts, skate shoes, hometown T-shirt. His friend, my
neighbor, was in his 50's and the bad-boy looked maybe ten
years younger. "Too old for me," I thought, and kept working.

That afternoon, I paddled out for my second session of the
day at the crappy little beach break 100 yards in front of my
300 square foot beachfront shack. I was just learning to stand
up on a surfboard. I had been bitten by the surf bug that
summer and was experiencing my first taste of its symptoms.
The waves were small but the wind was whipping as it
normally does in Southern California after 11 AM. I still
hadn't figured out how to read the rip current and my 8'6"
was far too big to duck dive even if I had known how. I
struggled to paddle out for 20 minutes. Without ever making
it out, completely defeated, I called it a day and headed back
for the beach. I saw my neighbor and the handsome bad boy
sauntering toward me, a longboard under one of his inked
arms.

"Kurt, Natasha. Natasha, Kurt." My neighbor made the
introduction.

"Howsitgoin?"

Kurt's clear, water blue eyes pierced me for a moment, then descended to inspect the sand.

On the pretense that we could surf together sometime, he asked for my number. He texted me within an hour.

There's a new surf movie on Netflix I want to see. Dinner at the Noodle House and movie later?

Uh-oh, that sounded like a date. I had just escaped a year-long relationship fewer than three weeks before. And before that, I had been married and still ugly. I was far from the end of my male attention binge, not yet satiated, not yet ready to be tied to one person. And he was too old for me, right? But Kurt's attention tasted good. What the heck, I thought. I could just add him to my growing list of friends with benefits.

Sure, sounds fun.

Later that night, sitting at the Ocean Beach Noodle House, I ordered a hot saki and Kurt ordered a Coke.

"You don't drink?" I was shocked.

"No, I haven't had a drink in three and a half years."

"That's weird," I remarked. Kurt explained to me that he had gone sober several years ago, after ending a 20 year battle with methamphetamine. *Oh, a man with issues, I can be of use!* My interest was piqued.

"The desire is completely gone. I don't mind if you drink in front of me. There's no way in hell I'm ever going back. It's like the old has gone and the new has come."

My ears perked up at his quoting of the Book of Revelations.

"Are you religious?" I asked.

"I believe a higher power has saved my life. I have a daily reprieve from my disease, contingent on the maintenance of my spiritual condition."

Every word increased his sex appeal. I didn't know he was quoting the Big Book of Alcoholics Anonymous. All I knew was that a man was buying me dinner, a man who had his shit together and valued spiritual growth. And that was hot.

Just before I met Kurt, I was going on dates with a few different guys. Now that I was single, all my male neighbors and guys I met surfing or at the gym suddenly wanted to know about my weekend plans. The attention was intoxicating. But Kurt was persistent. He wanted to see me nearly every day. I liked him a lot. I felt bad saying no to him. I didn't want him to think I wasn't interested and risk losing his attention or hurting his feelings.

One Friday night, I was pretty certain that I was rushing it too much with Kurt. I could see us heading toward a relationship--and I didn't want that. I was enjoying all the attention from other men and wanted to leave my options open. But instead of telling Kurt that I told him that I wasn't feeling like hanging out, and I was just going to do something with my neighbors.

My neighbors and I headed to a nearby bar that night. I spotted Dave at the bar. I had gone out with Dave a few times. He was fun enough, although I wasn't really interested in him. I hadn't seen Dave for a couple of weeks since meeting Kurt. Because I was always watching my weight, I was only drinking vodka soda that night. Dave bought me another one. The remainder of the night was mostly lost to a blackout. I've since learned that Vodka, even a small amount, causes me to blackout.

In the middle of the night, I woke up in Dave's bed. I was disgusted with myself. I considered myself to be "with" Kurt and had only wanted a little attention--not sex--from someone else. I keenly wanted to get out of there. I looked for my clothes but couldn't find my panties or belt. I didn't care, I just wanted to leave before he heard me. I threw on my dress and tiptoed out, running the six blocks home.

Consumed with self-loathing, I couldn't sleep. At the break of dawn, I grabbed my surfboard and paddled out. I saw Kurt in the water.

"How was your night?" he asked.
OMG, he knows! The guilt made me nauseous.

"Um, it was fun." My voice shook.

"How was Sunshine Company?" Another nausea-inducing question.

"How did you know I was there?" Panic shot through my chest.

"I figured you might be, since I know you like that bar. I stopped by to say Hi, but I saw you were with a friend."

"Oh, Kurt!" I blurted out, "I know that must have looked so bad. I'm sorry, I was all over him, I know!"

"But you didn't sleep with him? Because if we are not going to use condoms we have to communicate about this." He pronounced this with disturbing calm.

"No! Of course, not!" The lie came out of my mouth before I had a chance to think.

We agreed from there on out to be "exclusive". Kurt said he wasn't mad because we hadn't had the talk yet, but that he required 100% honesty from me moving forward. I agreed.

A week later, I was out of town on a business trip, scheduled to return home that night. Back at my apartment, Kurt had stopped by to drop off flowers for my arrival home. As he approached the door to my apartment, he spotted Dave exiting it. (I never locked my door). On the counter, next to where Kurt placed the flowers, lay a pair of my underwear, a belt, which Kurt recognized as the one I had been wearing that night, and Dave's business card. My phone started blowing up.

The rest of the work trip was brutal. I was so sick, I didn't eat. I rushed straight to Kurt's house upon returning home. I told him he should leave me that I had lied to him. I said I wouldn't be hurt if he could never see me again.

My panic increased when Kurt said he wanted us to read a prayer together. He forgave me and said he was 100% over it. This lie was supposed to be my ticket out. I knew I wasn't ready to restrict my sexual freedom. But Kurt forgiving me and being so spiritual about it made it impossible for me to acknowledge what I really wanted. What I wanted was to run around and be a slut. What I thought I needed was to be with a strong spiritual man. So, what I did is what good girls *should* do. I became monogamous...again.

Chapter 10: Never thin enough

As a beginner surfer, I was taking a lot of abuse in the beach break where Kurt and I liked to surf. As soon as I'd catch a wave I'd have ten more to deal with behind it, making my paddle back to the line-up very difficult. I didn't know yet how to read the waves and the rips to look for an easier paddle out spot. I didn't have strong paddling skills. I didn't know how to sink the back of my board with my feet in an up-dog position to make the front pop over the wave and then sink the front with my arms in a pushup position to make it back down the back of the wave. Learning to surf is the most exhausting part of a surfer's career. It takes a whole lot of stamina, determination, and willingness to fail.

Kurt was the kind of teacher who would rather put me in the right situation to figure it out for myself than to tell me how to do it. He said I needed to get to a point break. Having no clue what a point break was Kurt, drew me a diagram on a napkin over lunch one day. He explained how a finger of land would jut out into the ocean and the waves would break alongside of it, rather than toward it. He said this meant that at the end of a ride there would be a wide, deep water channel where no waves were breaking. I could paddle straight back to the top of the lineup without taking any waves on the head. This sounded good to me. And the idea of four days camping in the back of his truck on a deserted beach in Baja really piqued my interest. It sounded like a long craved adventure!

As we made the four-hour drive south of the border to Baja California, Mexico, Kurt depicted in great detail the 20-year battle he had fought with addiction. He recounted stealing money from his mom's purse, sleeping in his truck with no place else to go, getting high in the bedroom while he babysat his girlfriend's kids, going to every rehabilitation center in Southern California--and to some out of state centers too.

Finally, I asked, "Who is that guy you are describing? None of that sounds like the Kurt I know." His response seemed silly at the time.

"He's a monster. If I ever relapse, promise me right now that you will leave me. It won't be quick and it won't be easy. I would never want to put you through that. Promise me: if I ever relapse, you will leave me!"

I promised I would. And he promised it wouldn't come to that.

The next four days were not what I had hoped for. The water was frigid and the air not much better. I had only a cheap, entry-level wetsuit. No booties or hood. And I had so very little body fat.

As I have found many times before and after, the pleasure of my new relationship dulled the pleasure of food. My appetite was already weak due to the magic of being "fat-adapted", a state that I had worked hard to achieve. Constant attention from an older man and abundant, wonderful sex, made food almost unnecessary. My work was very slow at the time, so I devoted increasing stretches of time to exercise. The pounds continued to fall off. Over the course of four months, I reduced from a size 6 to a size zero.

I was 7-10% body fat. I knew, because I purchased test equipment and tested my composition almost daily. I still felt that my thighs were too big; I couldn't stand to look at them in the mirror. My body had started to cannibalize its own muscle for fuel. When a body reaches this point, it starts shutting down all non-essential functions. There simply isn't enough fuel in my body for digestion, emotional regulation, and proper hormone function.

We pulled up to the spot where the waves were breaking off a half-sunken ship which had run aground there decades earlier. There was no one else in the water, or anywhere for that matter. The waist to chest high waves were walling up for at least 100 yards, perfect for our longboards. There was no wind. The water looked like oiled glass. These are the conditions surfers dream of. Kurt rushed to pull on his wetsuit while I struggled to find the strength or motivation to get into mine. He told me to hurry. He said that at any time, five truckloads of people could pull up, the wind could shift or the swell could just drop. We had to take advantage of this perfect situation now while we had the chance.

I hardly made it 45 minutes before the cold became so painful even my bones hurt. Kurt surfed until well after sunset while I sat in the truck shivering and trying not to eat the crackers I had packed for him. Crackers have carbs. I wasn't allowed carbs. I ate two slices of cheese instead. Then I felt guilty. I wasn't exercising and I was just sitting there eating. I pulled on the warmest clothes I had and forced myself out of the truck for a jog up and down the point.

The trip was a success in that by the time we were ready to leave I had gotten at least half a dozen rides from the tip of the point all the way to the beach. My popup was improving and so was my paddle strength. Kurt said we should try to come back for the next big swell, mentioning something about the swell angle that went over my head.

As our relationship wore on, my surfing progressed in subtle increments so small I almost could not register them. But surfing continued to be my biggest source of joy, even as my energy continued to decline, along with my health. I would complain on the phone to my mom about how awful I felt: I was exhausted, I couldn't think, my digestion wasn't working and I picked up every cold and flu bug. I felt like I was dying because I was.

"I think you need to slow down a bit. Don't you think you are exercising too much?"

"Mom, the only thing that makes me feel better is exercise!"

"I'm worried you are going to have a heart attack though, honey."

"You are crazy, Mom! I'm just not feeling good, I don't have heart issues. I gotta go, it's almost sunset and I want to go for a run along the cliffs."

I hung up the phone and put on a hot pink sports bra, hot pink skin-tight shorts, size XS, and hot pink shoes. Just getting dressed exhausted me. I set off for a run along the cliffs, watching heads turn rather than watching the sunset. I made sure to run fast enough to pass any other girls out for a jog. I also made sure to notice who had thinner thighs.

Kurt's mother finally pointed out that I might have a problem with food. Kurt was befuddled at his mother's suggestion. He thought I looked great. He hated to see me feeling so crappy, so he suggested I give up running for a while and take up yoga. I agreed that something needed to change, since I didn't even have the energy to cook myself food. So, I joined a hot power vinyasa studio and took the most challenging classes offered, sometimes twice a day. But I didn't feel that yoga was a very good workout, so I would arrive early to do crunches and stay late to work on handstands.

I continued to refuse all carbs including, whole grains, fruit, and most vegetables. My weight continued to drop. My health issues worsened. I couldn't digest my food because my body was diverting energy away from digestion to maintain more essential functions. The food would sit in my stomach and rot. As soon as I ate, one of two things would occur: nausea, or an urgent need to run to the toilet. So commenced my bulimia.

It started innocently enough. I ate, I felt ill, I vomited, I felt better. I was, however, forcing the vomiting part by sticking a finger down my throat. But that was easy enough. Secretly, I loved the fact that eating made me feel sick. I could eat enough to satisfy the watchful eyes of those around me, then proclaim that I wasn't feeling well--which was true--and excuse myself to the bathroom. I fooled both myself and Kurt into thinking that my illness was physical instead of mental. The power of enjoying a meal without hours of painful nausea was addictive. Before long, I discovered that it didn't matter if I cheated on my diet or not. I was going to vomit it out anyway, so who cared what I ate?

During this time, I was working for a software company. The job required a great deal of travel on airplanes and a lot of overnight hotel stays. I arrived at my hotel late one night, exhausted and frail, as usual.

"What do you mean the elevator is broken?" I glared at the woman behind the front desk of the hotel.

"I'm very sorry ma'am, but we have just you on the second floor tonight and the stairs are right there."

That was all it took. Exhausted, I burst into tears right there in the hotel lobby. I turned around so I wouldn't embarrass myself. How could I explain that I was so entirely depleted that even the thought of walking up a flight of stairs made me cry? I made a scene of slamming down the retractable suitcase handle, knocking my bag on its side, and bending over awkwardly to hoist the bag off the ground by the side handle.

It might as well have been filled with lead. I could barely lift it to knee height. I teetered in my three-inch heels. My size zero pencil skirt restricted my thighs as I took tiny steps toward the stairs. Five stairs up, the edges of my vision went dark. I dropped my luggage and grasped for the rail, panting to catch my breath. My stomach churned. I felt like I was going to barf.

Eventually, I completed the odyssey to my hotel room. I found fruit and dark chocolate on the bar, beside a thank you note for being an elite hotel club member. I threw it all in the trash, lest I give in to the sinful temptation of carbohydrates. I had already eaten 1100 calories that day. The food tracker app on my phone told me my carb intake was at 17 grams. If I went over 20, I was in danger of being knocked out of ketosis. I had awakened that morning in a different city and had gone to the gym in a different hotel. I had given a presentation on my feet for 7 hours, dropped off my rental car, boarded a shuttle to an airport, got on and off a plane, took another shuttle to another rental car company, drove to this hotel, and in the morning I would go to the gym here and do it all over again.

I trudged through my nightly routine, adjusting the AC, closing the blackout curtains, choosing the firmness setting on the adjustable bed, and brushing my teeth. Standing over the bathroom sink, I spied the apple I'd thrown away peeking out from the trash. The trash bag was fresh. I could just give the apple a quick rinse and it would be fine. *NO! There are so many carbs in an apple! But the skin is pretty much just fiber. Fiber would help keep me full overnight with almost no calories. I could just eat the skin by taking shallow bites.* I reached into the trash, retrieved the apple, gave it a rinse, and sank in my teeth, just below the surface of the skin. I allowed myself an additional two bites of the sweet white flesh. Oh, the decadence, the aroma of its natural sugars, the way the flesh exploded in my mouth! My entire body sighed in pleasure. I took two more deep bites, filling my mouth with delicious sin.

Guilt. Sickness. Disgust. I had to get it out of me. *NO! It's just an apple. Don't puke! Go to bed.* But such lack of discipline is exactly how people end up fat and unhealthy. *Out! NOW! It has to come out!* But then another thought gripped me...*What about the chocolate?* If I was going to puke anyway, I might as well enjoy the chocolate first. I fished the chocolate out of the trash. It was gone in under 15 seconds. I was already leaning over the toilet before I swallowed.

I pulled back my hair, lifted the toilet seat, dropped to my knees, and inserted the index and middle finger of my right hand deep into my throat. I gagged once, twice, and there it was. First the frothy brown chocolate and then, still perfectly red, the skin of the apple came up looking the same as it went in. I made sure to look closely. Success! It hadn't had time to be broken down by stomach acids, which meant almost no calories had been absorbed. I flushed the toilet, washed the vomit off my face, rinsed my mouth, and went to bed. Tomorrow, I would wake up and do it all over again, and the scale would be none the wiser.

A friend suggested I see a therapist about my issues around body weight and fitness. I felt incredibly weak-willed. I felt like I had a problem controlling my desire to eat. I agreed that maybe a therapist could help--help me get control of my unruly appetite, that is. I met this particular therapist only one time. I don't remember her name or anything from the session, except when she took off her glasses, set down her pen, leaned in, and said,

"You have an eating disorder."

"Oh...no, I don't think I was clear. This isn't an eating disorder. I'm legitimately really hungry. I don't starve myself. I am just really good at sticking to a healthy diet. It's not like

I'm binging and purging. I only throw up when I feel nauseous. I don't have an eating disorder. I just feel ill. I just have a physical stomach disorder, not an eating disorder."

"Natasha," she leaned back in her chair and folded her arms, "you are paying good money for my professional opinion, and you can do with it whatever you want. But you DO have an eating disorder."

I never went back to see her again. I wish I could remember her name. I'd like to send her a thank-you note.

My risky relationship with food progressed and my health issues worsened. I had my hormone levels tested and discovered that I was in early menopause--at 30 years old. I had stopped producing the hormones needed for childbirth. I had tricked my body into thinking that I lived in a period of famine, that it was an unsafe environment in which to bring forth a child. Not only had I stopped menstruating, I was exhausted, had hot flashes, night sweats, aching joints, aging skin, and extreme emotions. I had, what seemed to me, a perfect-looking body. But I felt like a 65- year-old grandma. And, totally incapable of being honest with myself, I had no idea why all this was happening. I had seen several doctors who continually referred me to more doctors.

My first real wakeup call arrived during a work trip. I was battling a fever, but doing my job anyway. Late at night, I was driving to the hotel after my flight. I was too exhausted to think, my body too frail to fight the illness, and I made a mistake. At 60 mph, I swerved slightly off the road. My rental car struck a rock the size of a basketball. The tire blew out, the fender was smashed, and I got lucky. I knew what had happened was a result of exhaustion. I almost admitted to myself I was this very close call. Later that week, my fever would progress into the flu and, along with it, a urinary tract infection, bronchitis, and an outbreak of staph infection on my skin. My immune system lacked the energy to keep up with all these assaults. I was so ill that I feared for my life. In high school, I weighed 155 pounds. Now, at 117 pounds, my body was giving up. I admitted to myself that something was wrong.

My eating issues continued to create dangerous situations. One day, Kurt and a friend were going to surf a new spot. I was invited along. I was nervous. I felt like crap that day. In fact, I had been enduring a nondescript "crap" feeling for a number of months. At twenty-five pounds under my natural weight, I had no energy, my bones felt cold and the thought of getting off the couch and into the cold ocean made me a little nauseous. I knew surfing was way above my energy level, and that to surf while feeling the way I did was a great way to get hurt. But I hadn't yet had a workout that day, and no amount of crappy feeling was going to make me skip a workout! So, it was either surfing or high-intensity interval training. Surfing sounded a lot better.

Hoping a little sugar would pick me up, I threw an apple into my backpack along with my wetsuit, booties, and hood. Walking out the door, I second-guessed myself.

A whole apple? That's like 15 grams of sugar! That's going to knock me out of fat-burning mode! I'm going to store that in my liver, which means I'm going to store water with it. I've gotta weigh in tomorrow and that's definitely going to affect my number. No way! I'll just eat half.

I took out the apple, sliced it in half, and stuck it in a ziplock. My anxiety quieted, for the moment.

Kurt, his buddy, and I started on foot the one-mile-plus trek to the surf spot, hiking down a cliff face with nine-foot longboards. Then we marched across a beach, paddled around a point, crossed a second beach, and finally paddled another third of a mile out to the break. I was in agony before we even finished the hike down the cliff. Every cell in my body screamed for fuel. Finding none, my cells went searching for fat to burn. Certainly, no glucose was available for fuel, because I hadn't touched carbs in a year. And no body fat was available for fuel, either. So, my body resorted to cannibalizing its own muscle. Nitric acid was dumped into my system to burn muscle for fuel. It made me nauseous. But I attributed the nausea to having eaten the apple-- well, half an apple. Guilt from 7.5 grams of sugar made me want to puke.

As we filed along the cliff, Kurt's buddy eyed me, remarking "You don't look too happy..."

More guilt. What's wrong with me? Get it together! You are being given an opportunity few people ever get!

"I'm just tired today, but I'm stoked to surf," I lied, more to myself than to him.

By the time we reached the take-off zone, I was spent, mentally, and physically. I was nauseous, and the corners of my vision were black. With each paddling stroke, my shoulders screamed for me to stop. I shivered under my thick, 4/3 wetsuit, even though I had only been in the water for fifteen minutes. I paddled for four waves and missed each one, maybe because I was drained, but probably because I was scared. My subconscious knew that I was in no condition to survive a big wipeout, so at the moment for the last stroke, the stroke of do-or-die commitment, I backed off.

Mind over matter, I told myself, *your fear is holding you back, just GO!* I forced myself onto the next wave. I made it to my feet and for a split second felt victorious. But before I could savor the moment, my body, pushed to its limit, said enough is enough. My knees buckled, my board pitched forward and I somersaulted backward, toward the crashing white water.

Everything went black. Up became down as I spun like a sock in a dryer. A hot flash tore across my shoulder, but panic blocked the pain as I fought frantically to find my leash. The board, still attached to my ankle, rode on without me, dragging me underwater. I thrashed until I caught hold of the leash. My board stood upright like a tombstone on the surface, and I climbed the leash toward a second chance at life. I breached the surface, gasping for air. At the fourth breath, I noticed blood in the water. Although I felt no pain, my fragile body heaved with sobs. *What the fuck is wrong with you, you stupid bitch?* I was certain that I was an awful human being for taking such a huge wipeout. Humiliated, I let the white water push me to shore so I could calm down before going back out. The boys were still out. I should be out too.

Shivering, I hoisted my board and waded to the beach. I sat for a minute, mustering the courage to try again. I examined the board, feeling relief when I noticed a missing fin. A three-inch gash had been cut though my wetsuit and into my bicep. Pain throbbed and blood issued from my shoulder. I made the connection between the missing fin and the flash of heat I had felt as the wave expended her power on me. With a missing fin, there was no way I could continue my surf session. I was excused.

The boys continued to surf. I battled through the mile hike back out, dumped my board in Kurt's truck, and forced my tears to shut off. I reminded myself that shivering burns calories, as do physical and mental trauma, and walking. I proceeded to walk the additional two miles home, bleeding, shivering, exhausted, and alone.

My obsession evolved from simply not eating towards
"healthy" eating. I wanted to feel better so I assumed a
"cleaner" diet would do the trick. I started juicing, eating
superfoods and drinking chalky shakes. If it wasn't organic,
non-GMO, gluten-free and paleo, I was too good for it. There
is a clinical name for this type of eating disorder. It's called
orthorexia--an obsession with healthy eating. I controlled my
urges to binge and purge for months at a stretch, swearing
never to do it again. I refused to believe that I had a problem. I
convinced myself that I was just physically sick, which I was,
but I couldn't see that I was the cause of my own misery. I
read every blog about healing the gut and autoimmune
diseases, listened to podcasts on "bulletproof eating" and
"primal living". I paid hundreds of dollars a month for
supplements. As I started to be able to eat more food again,
my hunger returned, ten times stronger. And I started gaining
weight. Eating breakfast 3 times in a single morning and
puking up the last two became a daily ritual. I couldn't fight
the primal hunger, but I couldn't gain weight either...not after
I finally looked this good! I couldn't understand why I still felt
awful, drained of energy, constantly sick, and not getting my
period. I was slowly losing control of my body. I felt myself
slipping away and it terrified me. But control is like that. The
more you cling to it the painful it's eventual loss becomes.

Chapter 11: Repressed Desire Always Rises to the Surface

Midwestern farmer's granddaughters from homeschooling, evangelical Christian families are not allowed to have desires. We are wholesome. Singing in the choir, we are girls who can cook and clean and raise children. We are mild-mannered women who marry attractive, tall, white men with nice white-collar jobs. We live in homes we own. We drive cars we lease. We definitely do not have wants[E1] . We support our husbands in their work, stay quiet and suffer long. We put the needs of our families in front of our own. And, if we are ever honest enough with ourselves to feel a longing, we are even more miserable--because we certainly would never pursue it. That might inconvenience someone.

Because we have no idea how to say no, we assume no one else does either. So, we avoid asking for anything, as someone might say yes but not actually want to do the thing we've asked. We worry that asking will be too much of a bother and may cause someone to not like us. And what could be worse than not being liked? Then we will be lonely. Instead, we say what we don't mean, trying to make everyone else happy and ending up the loneliest people on earth. Women like me do not have the luxury of acknowledging desire. Better to learn to stop feeling it.

We become experts at talking in code, skirting the topic when we want something from somebody. In turn, we get really good at guessing what someone might want from us. We become chameleons with our words. And we become mind readers.

After a year of dating, Kurt and I got a place together--to my parents' keen dismay. After I informed my parents, we didn't speak for six months. They told me they loved me, but they didn't love my choices and could never support me in making my own decisions when I made such harmful ones. Of course not, because my values didn't mesh with theirs. How could anyone be different and be right at the same time? I misread their position as unconditional love. I didn't understand that it was indeed the definition of *conditional* love. And because this was my model for love, I practiced exactly this conditional love with my boyfriend. If he made me happy, I loved him. If he didn't, I claimed to love him, refused to leave him, and forced him to change.

Typical for a couple newly living together, issues emerged in our relationship. As we became more comfortable with each other, sweet loving acts dwindled and boredom set in. Kurt watched more television and spent less time with me.

Kurt's ambition for his new business faded and I jumped in, appointing myself the rescuer. I designed marketing materials and a website, and made appointments for him to bid on jobs. But he failed to follow through. Kurt simply lacked ambition. His values differed from mine. I loved him, but I didn't love his choices. It never occurred to me that someone might be a good person and yet have different values. I had no idea that I could let someone else be who they are, love them for it, and at the same draw boundaries and not allow that person to be an intimate part of my life. People were either bad or good. Good people organized their lives the way I organized mine. I believed Kurt was a good person, so I pushed him to become more like me. It didn't work.

Our relationship did not fulfill me. I had expressed my desire for him to be more ambitious, but nothing had changed. Advocating for myself and removing myself from the relationship wasn't something I had the strength to do. Plus the sex was good. I loved the roughness of it - being made the object of mad desire. It made me feel both powerful and worthless, like the worthless piece of shit my subconscious still believed I was, like the sexual goddess, capable of controlling a man, some deeper part of me needed to be. But somehow in the relationship, I didn't appreciate those same feelings. Feeling like I meant nothing to him, feeling that he was only with me for sex. An emotional connection, a sense of adventure, and a curiosity about the world were not present in our relationship. So I set aside my desires for a spiritually fulfilling relationship and assumed the role of martyr. *Look at me, living with this man so full of unrealized potential. Surely my suffering will save him.*

Just before I quit my corporate job, I cashed in on some vacation time, airline miles and hotel points, and booked us a trip to Hawaii. As surfers, we were ecstatic to visit the mecca of surfing, the North Shore of Oahu. Sitting on the plane, I leaned over to Kurt and told him there was something important I want to talk about. I'd been going to therapy. My therapist had stressed the importance of actually saying the things that make me feel like I'm choking. I had been feeling this awful tension in my chest for a couple of weeks. Finally, on the plane, I decided it was time to just speak.

I told Kurt I had been feeling more like a roommate recently. I told him I didn't feel significant to him. I told him I needed a little more affection. I said I wanted to see a little more ambition coming from him. He said he hadn't noticed anything and apologized. He asked if we could talk about something else and just enjoy the vacation. I didn't mention it again.

Two days later, standing in the rain on a beach in Hawaii, Kurt pressed a small box into my hand. Cracking it open, I hoped I was wrong about what I thought might be inside. Having already been married once, I really wasn't in a hurry to do it again. Plus, we had been having some new issues since moving in together.

The box held what I hoped it did not--a diamond ring. When Kurt asked those four words, tension gripped my chest, competing with genuine happiness and excitement. For a brief second, my heart urged me to say no. But how could I reject this man? It would be crushing to him. I didn't want to hurt him. In an instant, a plan sprang to mind. I would say yes, but we would be one of those couples who are engaged for years and never actually bothers with the wedding part. I said yes. I believed I could love him unconditionally and yet still want him to change, just like the example I had in Christ. Unconditional love, conditioned on following my rules.

We called my parents to tell them we were engaged. I was shocked when they were elated. To their minds, Kurt was finally going to make an honest woman of me after we had been "shacking up" for months. My parents suggested we get married ASAP. In fact, "Why not just do it while you are there in Hawaii?" they pushed.

Once again, happily ever after, the approval of my parents and God, and fulfillment of all the *shoulds* in my life, were all dangling just behind a quick ceremony on the beach. We were, after all, trying to start a business at the time, and weddings are expensive. My heart knew better but my mind still held the reins. So I bought a white bikini, and eight days later we eloped on Sunset Beach on the North Shore of Oahu. That morning we surfed tandem (two people on one big board) in Waikiki and that afternoon we exchanged leis, kissed, and posed for the camera. It was beautiful, the ocean was a spectrum of greens and turquoise, the sky was awash with blues and purples, his watery blue eyes locked on mine. I was finally doing everything right, and that meant everything would be perfect from here on out.

Addiction is a sneaky little bitch. The thing about recovery is that it requires constant vigilance. The Big Book of Alcoholics Anonymous says that the addict has a "daily reprieve" from his addiction "based on the maintenance of his spiritual condition." Meaning the addict is never healed but must maintain constant vigilance. It is true for non-addicts as well. People are either expanding or contracting. Everything we see, everything we eat, the way we spend our time, the people we surround ourselves with, the information we consume--it all has a vibrational value. When we consume things that vibrate at a higher frequency, we grow. But if the majority of the things we consume are at or below our current vibrational state then we are dying. For most people, these periods of lower vibrational consumption are when illness, depression, and financial problems sneak in. This is when people look for ways of escaping their low vibrations which include substances, television, and staying very busy. But an addict is not like other people. When an addict stops feeding his soul with positive energy, he will slip back into addictive behaviors.

Kurt felt he had arrived. He'd won a much younger, beautiful wife, a decent job, a nice place to live, and plenty of free time. His vigilance began to slip. His complacency would prove fatal to his sobriety.

Relapses happen long before the addict actually starts using drugs again. Positive behaviors lapse into neutral behaviors. Volunteer commitments, spiritual books, and exercise are replaced with TV and sleeping late. Positive friendships are replaced with dramatic, negative ones. Soon, even neutral behaviors slide into even lower energies; smoking, spending too much money, and skipping work to stay in bed. I could see it coming.

And I too was beginning to binge on lower frequencies. Worry, anxiety, and ego fed my racing thoughts even into my dreams at night. And I knew how to stop it. I knew all the right things for Kurt to do. He had to stop watching TV all day. He had to go to the gym. He had to put more effort into his business. He had to write down goals and make a plan on how to get there. He had to be of service more. And my suggestions would indeed have worked. But I wasn't saying anything he didn't already know. I arrogantly assumed he was ignorant of the healthy behaviors he needed to adopt. The reality was simpler: he didn't want to change.

I saw what I was doing. I had already been through the exact same break down in my previous marriage with Josh. I once created a folder on Josh's computer containing all the local activities for him to get involved in, from sports meet-ups to live music in order to draw him out of his depression. He deleted the folder without opening it and told me not to touch his computer.

This time, I refused to be the nit-picking wife. I shut my mouth and instead let all the thoughts about how I knew so much better than him build up in my head. I also refused to acknowledge that in order to have an equal partnership, I would need to be with someone who had different values. I was married. I had to take what I got. Eventually, I just shut up and let Kurt do his thing, silently blaming him for my own suffering. My vibrational energy dropped further and further. I kept myself ultra-busy at work, ignored bigger problems. My addiction was lying dormant just under the surface as well. Food issues grew larger and uglier.

Our household descended into near silence. Kurt would lie on the big couch watching surf videos, while I would lay on the small one, "wisely" using my time to complete work tasks on my computer or read personal development books. I silently judged him for not producing more with his time.

An expert from childhood at reading body language, I felt every subtext, each word lurking just beneath the actual conversation. I felt every flinch, pulling away, bristle, and cold shoulder. And it all felt the same. I felt everything, yet I could only feel one thing. I felt hungry.

My already starved body revolted in the face of this kind of anxiety. If I could not say what I meant then at the very least I wanted to hide the pain behind the pleasure of food. Each morning's first thought became, *What can I eat today that will fill me up but won't make me fat?* Thoughts of eating held my mind hostage, consuming nearly all my headspace. My animal brain fought for survival. But all I wanted to do was to stop being hungry. I spent countless hours researching the physiological causes of hunger and how to stop them. I tried every bio-hack on the internet, from fat-adaption to juicing to intermittent fasting. It didn't matter how much or little I ate. The tricks I had used before didn't work anymore. I was ALWAYS hungry.

I could feel my marriage slipping away. My old friends, Depression and Anxiety, surged back stronger than ever. The only action I knew to remove my discomfort was to eat. But gaining weight wasn't an option. The hunger was incessant. My unhappiness in my marriage was too scary to face. It was easier to blame my unhappiness on something more within my control: my weight. So the best solution to all of my problems seemed to be to control my insatiable appetite.

Kurt had become complacent. I became anxious, forcing my desire into the confines of my subconscious. I had an appetite for so much more out of life. And it showed up as physical hunger. Sitting at my desk, I would try to accomplish work, but thoughts of food crowded my brain.

Finally, ten years of starving myself with restrictive eating had caught up with me. This time, survival instincts triumphed over will power. There was no diet in the world that was going to work anymore. You can only repress what you really want for so long. I wanted to be nourished. My starved body seemed to move without my permission. I would indulge in a food I had labeled as "bad", or eat just enough calories so that I felt "bad". The black and white thinking I had inherited from the church activated. Suddenly, I was a bad human. Guilt converted minor indulgences into full-on binges.

I remember my first intentional binge. It was at the beginning of my workday. I checked my work email for the third time. I opened a PowerPoint that needed editing. I checked Facebook. I took a quick peek at my personal email. *Gosh, I'm hungry!* I ambled to the kitchen. My dirty breakfast dishes lay soaking in the sink. I gave a bowl a quick rinse, poured the day's second helping of granola, added some plain, non-fat, Greek yogurt, and returned to my desk. Munching, I clicked over to my work email, then back to the PowerPoint. I finger-scraped the remaining yogurt from the bowl and put the bowl next to my computer and began editing my presentation.

But the bowl was so gross and distracting, and my fingers were sticky. I carried the bowl to the kitchen and gave it a rinse. *Gosh, I'm still freaking starving!* I grabbed the box of granola and plunged my hand in. After eating two or three handfuls, I flipped the box to inspect the nutrition information. I didn't want to know. I set down the box. I picked it up. I set it down. I picked it up and carried it into my office and sat it next to my computer. An hour later, the box was empty, my Facebook status had been updated twice, my presentation still wasn't done, more emails had arrived in my inbox and I was still starving. Desperate to feel full, I speculated that maybe I hadn't consumed enough micro-nutrition. I found a banana, slathered it in almond butter, and devoured it. *Shit!* I was still hungry! *Maybe I hadn't had enough protein?* I opened the canister of protein powder and measured a scoop into a cup. *Darn, we're out of milk….Well, I need some more fat to feel satisfied anyway!* I mixed the powder with coconut oil and ate the concoction with a spoon. It was a little too dry, so I added a bit more oil. Then it was runny, so I added more protein powder.

Guilt. In my head, I quickly tabulated my sin: box of granola, 900 calories, yogurt, 250 calories, banana with almond butter, 300 calories, scoop of protein powder, 150 calories, 2 tablespoons of coconut oil, 250 calories...Ugh! I had just eaten my entire caloric allotment for the day, plus some. It was only 10:23 am...and I was still hungry.

Screw it! This has to come out. This has to come out! All of it out! I made up my mind that what was in my belly would have to come out. But then a thought struck...I had already screwed up, I was already about to make myself vomit, why not just feel full for a few moments of pure bliss before I pay the penalty for my sin?

Like coffee jitters, anxious panic shook my body. My hands flew from cupboard to fridge to freezer and back again, looking for something I could eat. I didn't want Kurt to get suspicious, so I decided just to eat a little of everything. The more "bad" I had deemed the food, the more I enjoyed it. Two pieces of bread with almond butter, 4 Triscuits, a scoop of ice cream, a little more ice cream, a handful of nuts, a bite of a chocolate bar from the freezer, a little of last night's leftovers.

The food went in faster and faster. I chewed less, tasted less, and swallowed more. I careened from sweet to salty, from cold to hot and back again. Each bite brought a tiny hit of dopamine and each swallow a feeling of loss. I wanted more, more, more! I checked every cupboard, the fridge, and freezer. I checked them again. Anxiety gripped me when I realized I could eat nothing more without arousing suspicion. I sped to the bathroom.

Hair in a ponytail, toilet seat up, knees on the ground, fingers down throat. I watched as my sins were punished in reverse order: leftovers, then ice cream, followed by nuts, bread, and finally granola. I gagged one last time, trying to rid myself of any final calories. I rose, washed my face, cleaned the toilet bowl, brushed my teeth, and returned to my computer. Exiting the bathroom, my entire body relaxed. For the next two hours, I rode the calm; my PowerPoint was completed and emailed, and I was onto my next task before I knew it.

Two more binges took place that week. Over the next couple of months, the frequency of my binges increased and the amount of food I ate during each binge increased as well. I hated it. I didn't want to do it. I knew how unhealthy it was. But I was starving, all day, every day, constantly wanting to eat but denying myself until all my willpower was spent. The only time I wasn't thinking about food was within that brief window of euphoria immediately following a binge. I hated feeling so helpless.

A binge feels like the ultimate Fuck It. *Fuck feeling this way, fuck being skinny, fuck what I'm supposed to do, fuck the food rules. I'm fucking hungry and I'm going to fucking eat.* At least that's how it starts. That is the animal inside, struggling to survive at all costs.

But once the rules are broken, the first forbidden food consumed, I want to stop. I really do. And I do stop. Chewing stops, swallowing stops, I set down the empty container. And

I feel sick. *What have I just done?* The guilt-induced nausea intensifies the longer I am still. There are two ways to stop the sick feeling: I can vomit or I can eat something flavorful enough to overpower the guilt. For a moment, I can distract myself with decadent chewing, slurping, tasting, and swallowing.

But I knew I shouldn't purge. The only options seemed to be chocolate or ice cream or chips or--most typical for me-- protein powder mixed with coconut oil. There was nothing else "bad" in the house, but each time the chewing ceased, when the flavor had left my tongue, after I had swallowed, the nausea returned, and stronger. Three more bites, a momentary pleasure, yet more nausea. I ranged from concoction to concoction, each one richer and sweeter than the last. Each time I finished a dish, a feeling of loss filled me, soothed only by yet another bite. My body fought to live, and I struggled to be thinner.

A binge is awful. And I hated doing it. So I started reading eating disorder books. They suggested that I ate to fill some emotional need. I hated this idea. It was the most idiotic thing I had ever heard. The books suggested that I try to comfort myself in some other way, like taking a walk. Bullshit! I was hungry, fucking hungry! I was hungry for food, for sex, for emotional connection with my husband, for a fulfilling job. No fucking walk around the block was going to cure me. But all I felt was the need for calories, more and more calories.
I went to see a new therapist, this time semi-admitting that I had a problem in my relationship with food. She suggested I pay attention to the emotions I was feeling just before a binge. Emotions? I was HUNGRY, really, really fucking HUNGRY. I didn't know anything about any emotions. All I knew was that I was hungry and, no matter what, I wasn't going to get full.

Finally, I stumbled upon a book which explained *scientifically* what happens to the brain after prolonged extreme caloric restriction. The author explained that a starved body continues to feel starved, even after proper feeding, due to hormonal disruption, adding that the only way to reset the metabolism is to increase caloric intake dramatically. I had been starving and underfeeding myself for over a decade. My body was throwing a protest rally. The book prescribed eating until you were full. It said that you should expect to gain a significant amount of weight at first, but that eventually, the body restores itself to its set point. I felt vindicated. All of these years, books, therapists, group meetings...at last, I wasn't crazy or not dealing with my emotions or battling childhood traumas. I was fucking hungry. But I couldn't possibly eat as much as I was hungry for. I would gain weight. I could imagine no worse fate. So I continued to find myself kneeling on piss-covered floors in gas station bathrooms, my fingers down my throat and vomit in my hair. Nothing could be worse than getting F.A.T.

Chapter 12: F.A.T.

Two years into the relationship, Kurt and I were both holding on by a thread. I ignored him as I spent long hours building my yoga brand, and he ignored me while spending long hours watching TV. Eventually, the tight feeling in my chest returned, and we revisited the conversation we'd started on the plane...the conversation we'd started just a few days before I agreed to spend the rest of my life with him.

One night, sitting on opposite couches, Kurt zoned out to the TV while I browsed my email. The silence was so loud I couldn't take it. I was going to say what needed saying for years but I had been too scared to admit to myself even existed. The familiar tension in my chest seemed to choke me. I gathered all my courage. I blurted out that I was feeling like a roommate, not a lover, that sex had dwindled, that he didn't compliment me or touch me anymore, and that I felt like I annoyed him more than anything.

"Well, there is one thing we should talk about," he said. He muted the TV and asked me to come sit by him. He looked me in the eye and said words I will never forget.

"I love everything about our relationship. I have so much fun with you. I really love you."

He rested his hand on my leg. I could feel him setting up to dish out a blow.

"There is just one problem," he paused to choose his words, "You've gained so much weight, I'm just not attracted to you anymore."

I wanted to puke. My entire body, not just my stomach, felt

like it was going to vomit. My blank face refused to form an expression. I was motionless. Time stopped. Finally, I managed to say that I didn't understand. He clarified.

"Well, you have gained a lot of weight since the wedding."

"I've gained three pounds."

It was true. I tracked my weight weekly, with an app. I had gained three pounds. I had six-pack abs and rope-like arms. My veins popped out of my forearms. I wasn't getting my period because I was underweight for my frame.

But I knew exactly how he had arrived at the idea that I was getting fat. I had given it to him myself. He knew my biggest vulnerability. He was subconsciously choosing to exploit it.

My body was as lean as ever, yet my body image was in the worst shape. I constantly complained about how I felt fat. The complaining was really just my way of looking for reassurance that I was not fat at all, or that, even if I was fat, I was still loved. But no outside source could ever give me the validation I needed. What I was asking from Kurt was not only unfair, it was impossible for him to give. To make matters worse he was unhealthier than ever, having nearly stopped all of the practices he regularly kept tostay sober. He knew exactly what to say to cut at me deepest. He too was looking for a way out of an unsatisfying situation.

I grabbed my purse and my journal and left. I spent the night in the yoga studio. After two hours of crying in child's pose, I remembered the warning Kurt had given me when we first started dating:

"If I ever relapse, promise me you will leave me."

It was a loophole to my vows on Sunset Beach. I told my journal, *I want out. A part of me hopes he relapses. Of course, I don't want that for him, I just want out.* I thought of how I would scan Josh's computer for porn, waiting for him to give me justification to leave him. Good Christian girls don't just give up on marriage. I would need a better reason than just being miserable to get out. I piled up ten yoga mats and used two more for blankets. I spent a sleepless night tossing my bony frame from side to side and crying, feeling absolutely trapped.

The next morning, I told Kurt something had to change. He promised that things would change. He promised he would go to more meetings, go to therapy, meet with his sponsor, sponsor other guys in the program. And he meant it. He felt awful. He really did love me, but we shared the same issues, and neither of us loved ourselves.

We both tried. We both went to therapy, I attended my recovery meetings for food and he attended more of his own meetings. We weren't fighting--we never fought. But fighting would have been better than the silence we inhabited. At home, I walked on eggshells, a big lump in my throat preventing me from speaking. Sitting on the big couch, Kurt zoned out to the TV. I sat on the small one, both ten feet and a million miles away. He watched shows about people fishing for crabs in the freezing cold ocean, and I read books about eating disorders. I read them on my phone, so he didn't know what I was reading. Each night we sat in silence, distracting ourselves with TV and a book. In this way, we avoided having to ask the elephant towering between the two couches to please move.

Why are endings so scary? I had been playing the role of a loving partner for so long that revealing my true unhappiness would have been akin to uncovering some deep dark secret.

Dear lover, I haven't liked you since the first time the television took you away from me. I should have mentioned it that first night when the TV came on and I got shut out. But I went along with it even when it bothered me. Now it was too much to bear. Voicing my dissatisfaction surely would have meant the end of us.

Instead of making myself big enough to speak the truth, I made myself smaller. I made my needs smaller. I made my voice smaller. I made my body smaller. I was simply too big for Kurt to handle. I was too big to be with a man who was making himself so small. The more he regressed into himself, the smaller I needed to become. After all, I had promised God that I would not leave this man. At any cost to myself, I had to make the marriage work. I couldn't bear the thought of a second divorce.

A countless string of similar evenings in our household began to feel like Groundhog's Day. I cooked dinner, serving myself half of what I really wanted. We ignored each other, ignored our food, and watched TV instead. After dinner, I'd volunteer to clean up. This move bought me time out of sight in the kitchen to shove food into my mouth. Always still hungry, I was too afraid to eat seconds in front of Kurt.

Kurt spent the remainder of each evening under the spell of television. I can't stand TV and my brain couldn't tolerate the stillness, so I'd crack my laptop to do some research as he melted his brain away, his body itself melted into the big couch. Of course, he sensed my judgment, whether he was conscious of it or not.

My research topics on those lonely evenings were always related to "health". I desperately searched the internet for answers. My search queries varied widely, but the question was always the same: *How can I be thin and not constantly hungry, tired, and out of energy?* Link after link, I clicked deeper and deeper into despair. Each night I'd retire to the bedroom with a head full of new diet requirements.

I'd lay in bed and consider foods for the next day. I'd tally the calories in my head. I no longer needed a calorie tracker app, for I had memorized all the values. I'd hear the TV drone on and on from the other room. Kurt was turning his brain into mush, whereas I was using my time much more "productively". My stomach would rumble, still unsatisfied. I was experiencing symptoms of severe irritable bowel syndrome. My strange eating behaviors had thrown my gut biome so off-kilter that I now had trouble processing almost any food. My stomach would swell up and gurgle, gas filling every nook and cranny. When the gas started to release, I was very thankful that Kurt was not yet in bed with me. Months later, he confessed the reason he stayed on the couch so late every night. It was because of the stench in the bedroom. I had reached a new and deeply embarrassing low.

When my alarm sounded in the morning, my first thoughts were always the same. *What am I going to eat today that won't make me gain weight? How can I make this hunger go away without getting fat?*

I'd sit on the toilet for as long as it took, optimizing my use of time by reading an inspiring spiritual text while waiting for my body to feel a little less constipated. Then I'd strip off all my clothes and step on the scale. I looked forward to this brutal daily ritual. There was something sick about how much I loved this bashing. Like a powerful CEO going to a dominatrix for sexual pleasure, I mounted the scale each morning to savor my daily punishment. Numbers would flash onto the scale, giving me precise permission to treat myself like trash. Because, clearly, I *was* trash. Those numbers may as well have been the words, "Disgusting Bitch" or "Worthless,

Worse than Worthless, Nasty." Still echoing from my retinas, I carried those numbers with me into the kitchen. I prepared coffee and a breakfast of 350 or fewer calories. To fight off the craving for a second helping of breakfast, I reminded myself how awfully I was failing at life. I leveraged the number to pry myself out the door, packing just two boiled eggs for my lunch.

If the numbers happen to be lower, I would nevertheless conduct the same merciless under- eating regimen, but with a sense of anticipation and joy. I would reach for cream to add to my coffee, but think better of it; skinny girls don't need cream. I would dash carefree from the house without eating a thing. Hungry is the feeling thin!

Constant hunger became unbearable. The binges and purges were regular and frequent. I simply could not live with it any longer. I embarked on a mission to end it. I turned to self-help books once again.

The first book I read personified the "voice" of an eating disorder in the form of a guy named ED. Supposedly, ED lived in my head and persuaded me to eat like a starving person and then throw it all up. But I didn't hear any voices. I simply felt hunger. It didn't sound like a voice, it sounded like my stomach.

The next book enumerated some very simple food rules. Eat *only* when you are hungry. Eat *if* you are hungry. Eat what you are truly hungry for. These were the stupidest things I'd ever read. The author suggested that most hunger is emotional, and that if you eat only when you are physically hungry, then you won't overeat. That was a complete load of crap. I was physically hungry, weak, shaky, low energy, and starving ALL.THE.TIME. For me, if I ate when I was hungry, I would rapidly grow obese.

The third book was so far out there that I couldn't even finish it. It suggested that I follow my intuition, eating whenever my body told me to eat. Yeah, right! And turn into a 300-pound blob? NOPE!

The other books gave strategies for feeling emotions and dealing with stress. Check the mail or walk around the block when you feel a binge coming on. I tried it. I felt like binging, so I went for an eight-mile run. When I came back, I ate all the food in the house, vomited it up, bought more food, and vomited again. This variation on the strategy seemed to fall outside the scope of the book's recommendations.

The books contained all kinds of unhelpful suggestions. Take three deep breaths. Write a letter to your emotions. Call a friend to discuss what's bothering you. What was bothering me was that I was fucking starving. How the fuck was calling a friend going to make me less hungry?

The most laughable strategy of all, which seemed to appear in every single book, was taking a hot bubble bath. One night after dinner, I lay on the couch starving, reading my self-help books. I read about taking a bubble bath for the 17th time. I decided to give it a try. I filled the tub and added the suds. I lit candles and got comfy. Within two minutes, the only thing I could think about was how hungry I was. I tried to feel the warm suds on my skin and send love to my body like the books suggested, but my hunger kept hijacking my thoughts. The bath wasn't working. I started to cry. I was willing to do anything, but none of it made any sense. I felt helpless and hopeless.

I got out of the tub, toweled off, and stood on the scale. Up two pounds.

"FUCK YOUR FUCKING BUBBLE BATH!" I shouted at no one.

"You okay?" came the response from the next room.

"Yeah," I replied, and then quietly added, "Just really fucking hungry."

Of course, I was. At that point, I'd been chronically underfed for several years. Even after a large meal, I was still hungry. I was like the grumpy old penny pincher who had millions of dollars in the bank but, because he lived through the Great Depression, was scared to spend a dime. My body lived in constant fear of starvation because my life was full of fear and distrust of nature itself.

One day, I took a hammer to my scale. Three weeks later, I bought a new one. Another day, I had a friend hide my scale and I couldn't find it for weeks. Then, I stepped on a scale at someone else's house. I left her party early because I couldn't stand to keep my fat disgusting self around happy people. As my purges became more frequent, I started finding new ways of hiding them. Since my work was less than a mile from home, I often made an excuse to make a quick stopover in the evening just so I could use the bathroom without the risk of being heard.

I punched in the keycode and swung open the door to my yoga studio. Jasmine incense from a class earlier in the day wafted out. Wind chimes tinkled a gentle greeting. I closed and locked the door behind me. Removing my shoes, I entered the sacred studio space. Light streamed through etched glass windows to reflect from large mirrors, spreading into minute rainbows within the room. The serenity and healing ambiance of the studio contrasted starkly with the hurried path I cut to reach the bathroom on the other side of the studio.

Twenty minutes earlier, I was eating dinner at home. I was so hungry that I couldn't stop myself. A second helping turned into a third. An additional several bites found their way into my mouth as I put away the leftovers. Guilt overwhelmed me in a rush. I had to get this food out of me. But my husband was in the next room with two friends, watching surfing on the TV. The bathroom was adjacent to the couch; they would hear me for sure.

"I'm going to meet Kim for a walk," I called to Kurt, my keys in my hand. "I won't be gone long."

I ran to my car and dodged traffic on the 0.7-mile commute to my yoga studio. I ran mindlessly across the street to the gas station to buy a giant cookie. I shoved the cookie into my mouth as I approached the front door. I hustled past the windchimes, past the incense, past the streaming light and the dancing rainbows, and into the bathroom. I spit the half-chewed cookie into the toilet before I could swallow it and proceeded to dispose of my dinner as well.

When I finished, I washed my face with fancy, all-natural soap at the bamboo waterfall sink. I pulled out my phone and texted Kim to see if she had time for a walk, and she instantly texted back.

Actually, I'm walking by the studio now, I'll come grab you.

Shit! Guilt twisted my insides and I dug through the supply cabinet, frantically looking for toilet bowl cleaner to hide evidence of my sins before she arrived.

On another morning, I woke up ravenous--as usual. I made my bulletproof coffee, adding extra fat to keep me filled up during the workout I was to lead that morning. I downed the fatty coffee and still felt wolfishly hungry. I cracked an egg into a sizzling pan. It looked really small, so I cracked another one, and then a third. I doused them with hot sauce in order to force me to eat them slower. But it didn't work. I slurped them all down in under a minute.

I grabbed my water and purse and searched for my keys. As I reached the door, my hunger was out of control. I turned to face the fridge, *maybe just a few carbs to give me some fuel for my workout.* I opened a yogurt and ate it with my finger on my way to the car. I pulled up to the yoga studio and ran across the street to a 7-Eleven. *Don't do this, Natasha!* But my feet seemed to move themselves. I filled a 20 oz cup from the cappuccino machine and squirted as much whipped cream on top as the cup could hold. I sipped down the whipped cream as I examined the rack of protein bars. I grabbed a low carb protein bar and headed for the counter. But then I stopped, pivoted, and loaded more whipped cream onto my cappuccino before securing the lid. The protein bar was half gone before I even crossed the street.

Suddenly, I felt full. My appetite had finally been satisfied. And I felt miserable, disgusting, and ugly. I unlocked the yoga studio and glanced at my watch. I had 9 minutes before the girls would show up. I walked into the mirrored room and lifted my shirt. Sure enough, my belly was fatter today than yesterday. I started to cry.

No way, fuck this! I burst into the bathroom, lifted the toilet seat, put my hair up, dropped to my knees, stuck my index and middle finger down my throat, and gagged repeatedly. Protein bars were always hard to get back up, and the low carb kind was really sticky. I kept gagging until a vomity version of the bar appeared, floating in the toilet within frothy whipped cream. I plunged my fingers deeper until a coffee and egg mixture made its way up too. I flushed twice. I grabbed the toilet brush and cleaned up the mess on the backside of the bowl. I washed my face and made sure my waterproof mascara hadn't run.

"Hello?" Someone called from the lobby.

SHIT! Did she hear me in here? How long has she been here?

"I'm in the restroom, be right there!" I called back, injecting a fake smile into my voice. *I can't do this anymore. How many people am I lying to now? How many more people will end up with their face in a toilet bowl because of me?*

On a girls' trip to Baja, I got drawn too deeply into the peanut butter. We all brought our favorite snacks and spread them out on the counter in the big beachfront house. All the other girls dipped a chip or two into the salsa, got themselves into their bikinis, and went down to the beach. As soon as I was alone in the kitchen, I felt as if I was starving. But the chips and cookies were too unhealthy. I reached for an unopened jar of peanut butter.

Peanut butter is the hardest food to regurgitate. It's a bulimic's worst nightmare. And it is one of my all-time favorite foods. I love and hate peanut butter.

Eating in secret is the worst. I feel like there is something wrong with me because my body always seems to want more food than the other girls want. Of course, there is something wrong with me--I'm fat! I'm the fat girl with the full plate, while the popular pretty girls sit over there pecking at their carrot sticks. I feel like something is broken in my biochemistry. Some hormone that regulates hunger in hot girls is cranked up to 10 in my body and stuck there. All the other girls have their hunger hormones set at 3 with an auto-off feature that kicks in when they eat a piece of broccoli.

After devouring my peanut butter (and banana) treat I was instantly disappointed. A first ting of panic struck. That wasn't enough food. I'm still hungry. But that's already too many calories. That's more than any of the other girls ate. But I want more. But there are only two bananas left. If I eat another one, everyone will know! But I can't sit with this intense hunger. It is going to destroy me. It's too powerful. I'm too miserable. I have to eat!

I grabbed a cookie and fled the room, tapping all my willpower to do so. I changed into my bikini and avoided the mirror. As I left my bedroom, cookie long gone, the kitchen called me back. I stood at the front door, frozen. Wanting with all my will to just exit the house but unable to move.

Before I knew it, my feet were moving without my permission. My hands were reaching for the peanut butter, my mouth was licking and chewing. I made sure to hide the banana peel under some other trash so no one would see it. With my urges satisfied, I calmly joined the other girls at the beach.

Just before bed, one of the girls brought the snacks back out. We each dipped two pita wedges into hummus and called it a night. My stomach was growling. The M&M soft batch cookies looked so good. But I couldn't possibly. I noticed the only other girl who ate any cookies was the chubby girl on the trip. And even she ate only one.

I laid in my bed thinking only of peanut butter. I could see in my head exactly where the jar sat on the kitchen counter. I knew I was too hungry to sleep. I hated myself for being hungry. I hated that I had this crazy obsession. If hunger were located at a specific point in my body, I would have taken a knife to it and cut it out, no questions asked.

The peanut butter won. This time on pita bread because I didn't want to eat all the bananas. But I didn't want to eat all the pita bread either, so I just started dipping my spoon into the jar for a tiny bit more, a tiny bit more, a tiny bit more. Until...FUCK, over half the jar was gone. I panicked. I couldn't eat anymore. There was nothing more to eat without eating all the snacks for the entire weekend. Hunger still gnawed at my insides, but I had to be done!

I knew there was only one way to turn off the madness. Purging is more powerful than Xanax for calming my anxiety. I was lucky because I had my own bathroom, away from the other girls. I could vomit in peace.

But it wouldn't come up. I gagged and sputtered. I stuck my finger deeper. I coughed and spit. But nothing came up. I could feel a big sticky peanut butter lump stuck halfway up my throat. I tried harder and harder. I drank water and tried again. Nothing. I gagged until my face hurt. Then I gave up. I went to bed fat, disgusting, miserable, and hungry.

The next morning, the first thing the girls said to me was, "Oh my god! What happened to your eye?" I had no idea what they were talking about. I checked my eye in the mirror. Half of it was blood red.

"I was crying a lot last night about my marriage," I lied, "I guess I burst a blood vessel from crying too much."

The guilt of living a lie was almost as awful as the idea of the fat I would have to gain in order to fix this problem. I knew being honest would mean ending the purging and restriction, which would mean gaining weight, which would mean ending my career in the fitness industry, ending my marriage, the ending of who I thought I should be. And I couldn't bear to entertain the thoughts. Not yet, the pain hadn't gotten bad enough.

When a child's caregiver is too busy to listen, the volume and shrillness of the child's requests will intensify until the child has become annoying enough that she cannot be ignored. Health issues are the soul's loudest, most annoying cries for help. Unfortunately, I have habitually failed to listen to the soft requests my heart makes, hearing it only when it shrieks impatient demands.

My bulimia was causing me gas and severe bloating issues. Constant binging and purging had created an imbalance of healthy gut bacteria, an extremely delicate and difficult condition to fix. I bought expensive and ineffective probiotics. Then I invested in methods for making my own probiotics: a yogurt maker, a kombucha setup, a sauerkraut crock. I bought digestive enzymes and learned ways to produce my own enzyme concoctions through juicing. I bought a juicer and spent a fortune on organic local veggies. I bought superfood tablets and powders, dehydrated seaweed and berries. I have no idea how much I spent monthly on all the supplements, juices, and probiotics, not to mention all the alternative healers I was seeing...but it was in the hundreds of dollars per month. Every time I forked over another wad of cash, a gnawing sensation in the pit of my stomach would insinuate, *You're doing this to be skinny*. But the message never spoke loudly enough for me to hear it. I suppressed its truth, reminding myself that I was sick and needed to get better...so I could get skinnier...*Oops, did I just say that?*

One day, I swore I would do whatever it took to fix this problem. I wandered around my neighborhood wearing Kurt's XL T-shirt to hide my painfully swollen belly. I ached with gas pains. I looked eight months pregnant. Walking and sipping green tea brought moderate relief. I walked for two hours, returned home, made more tea, and resumed walking.

My health issues worsened until, at last, sitting on crinkly white paper, perched on a table in another doctor's office, I hit my eating disorder bottom. I had endured the University of California San Diego hospital for more than three hours that afternoon. I had been to the lab twice to get needles stuck in my veins. I had seen four different doctors and three different nurses. Each specialist had entered, chatted with me, ordered labs, and returned with results. My labs showed I was sick, but the doctors and nurses couldn't figure out why. Finally, the fourth doctor strode into the room and shut the door behind her. She was in her second year of residency at UCSD. She was beautiful, thin, younger than me, wearing heels and a white coat. She sat down and didn't even bother beating around the bush.

"Natasha, have you ever had bulimia?"

My instantaneous tears answered for me. I made the decision at that moment never to make myself throw up again.

But I had no idea how much work that decision would require of me.

Chapter 13: An Excuse to Leave

I collected car trash while I waited for the pump at the gas station. I noticed a folded piece of paper sitting on the passenger floorboard. I opened it to find a receipt from a Motel 6 in Big Bear, California. A few days earlier, Kurt and I had traded cars for a weekend. I was leading a yoga and surf retreat in Baja, and needed his truck to haul surfboards. He needed my car and its snow chains for a snowboarding trip in the mountains. Kurt was edgy and withdrawn after the weekend, but I didn't question it. The receipt made no sense. Kurt always stayed at a friend's house when he went to Big Bear. My heart raced. I stopped myself before my mind could make up any stories. I picked up the phone and called him. No answer. I called again. No answer. I texted him, and there was no reply.

I knew it had been Kurt's old habit to rent a sleazy motel room to get high in, because he told me about it. But it had been nearly seven years since the last time Kurt got high. I couldn't let my mind go there. Was there another woman? I couldn't let my mind go there either.

Hours passed. Kurt always responded promptly. I texted some of his friends and his mom, but no one had seen him or heard from him all day. It was well past the time he normally came home from work. I could feel myself pushing down panic. Out of desperation, I called one of Kurt's sober friends whom he had known since childhood. Brock, a 25-year sober alcoholic, picked up the phone. I explained the situation: Kurt was missing, I found a hotel receipt from last weekend, he should have been home hours ago.

"Okay," he paused and sighed, "...I'm so sorry, sweety. Kurt is getting high right now. This is what he does. Call a girlfriend to be with you. He'll show up in a few days."

I will not forget that moment, one of a handful of moments in my life when my entire world shattered. I was driving, descending from the top of a hill on Narragansett street. It was evening, the sun setting. I hit the brakes, pulled over the car, thanked Brock for his help, hung up the phone, and watched my life fall apart.

Complete helplessness feels a lot like a big wipeout. It's black and cold and you don't know which way is up. You choke and fight for life, but there is nothing or no one to fight against, so you fight yourself, making matters worse, increasing the length and severity of the beat down. The wave doesn't let go, stronger than you will ever be. There you are, searching for something, anything, to cling to. And the wave continues to drill you. But the one thing you want to do more than anything in the world, to open your mouth and breath, is one thing that will kill you. To fight is to die. You must stay calm and rational, your life depends on it.

I returned to our empty home. Utterly helpless, I wanted to control something, anything. First I ate, I ate everything, until I was sick. Then, energized by vomiting--the ability to control my body when I felt so out of control--I had an idea. I knew how to find him. I knew the password for his iCloud account. I could log into the computer and trace his phone using the "Find my iPhone" feature.

I traced him to a grimy motel a few miles away. I called my friend, Kelsey. She was always up for some drama. She was also the only friend I knew would keep my secret and never judge me. Kelsey suggested we go get him. She came to pick me up, and we followed the GPS location. Sure enough, we spotted his truck in the parking lot. The hotel clerk would not give me the room number, so we waited outside the building.

I have no idea what we were waiting for or what we hoped to find or what we were going to do when we found it. I just knew that doing something felt better than feeling everything. I didn't want to feel anything.

"All this drama is giving ME anxiety," Kelsey declared as she pulled out a cigarette and lit up.

"Give me one of those!"

I had never really smoked much and it had been years since my last cigarette. The first drag made me sick to my stomach. And it felt good.

The next day, I couldn't trace Kurt's phone anymore; it must have died. Searching for control, I broke into his online bank account using his password and transferred all of his money into his savings account, so he couldn't access cash at an ATM nor purchase another night at a hotel. My emotions ran wild. I tried teaching a couple of yoga classes. For sixty minutes, I was able to shut down my personal world and pop into Teacher World. The classes were mechanical and rigid. They sucked. I called a sub for my evening class. I made plans to meet some business associates for a networking event that evening at a brewery. I couldn't allow myself to feel any of this, so I would pretend it wasn't happening.

As the day wore on and I distanced myself from my emotions, a new feeling came over me. Relief. I'd felt this particular relief once before, when Josh told me he was still using porn and that our marriage was over. I would feel it once more, when a business coach told me it was time to sell my yoga studio. Kurt's words came back to me.

"If I ever relapse, promise me you will leave me. Promise."

This was it, my ticket out.

I walked into the brewery that evening and made up my mind. I was out, it was over. Whenever he did come back, I was leaving.

Twenty minutes into my networking meeting, my phone buzzed. It was Kurt. I stepped outside to take the call.

"I relapsed." He was crying.

"I know." I started crying too. *Go away stupid tears!*

"I'm so embarrassed; I don't want you to see me like this."

"Come home now."

I couldn't understand why these words were coming out of my mouth. *C'mon Nat, stay strong.* But my will melted at his tears.

"Come home. Please, come home!" At that moment, I couldn't bear to hurt him any more than he was already hurting.

By the time I met him at home, it was late. He'd bought a six pack with him to help him come down from the drug high. I had never seen him drink. I kissed him. He tasted like beer. He tasted like all my exes before him. He wanted to call a drug counselor whom we both knew. He and Kurt used to serve together on a board at a recovery facility. Kurt wanted to check himself in. We called, and the counselor said he would be right over. The two of them talked while I listened with folded arms and a straight back. Kurt said he hated what he had just done and he never wanted to do it again. The counselor turned to me and asked what I wanted to do.

"I'm out. I'm filing for divorce tomorrow."

I had regained my will. My announcement rendered both of
them speechless. Neither of them had met this woman before.
This woman was strong and had a voice. The counselor urged
me to give Kurt thirty days. But Natasha-with-balls said No
Way.

Kurt was shocked. How could one instance of not coming
home merit divorce? His shock was justified. I had been
voiceless, unable to express how miserable I had been for
several months.

Kurt looked at me, his water-blue eyes glistening, and begged
me to give him thirty days. I heard Natasha, Kurt's wife,
agree. Thirty days. Then I was out. The part of me that didn't
know how to speak hoped he wouldn't make it. That part of
me was tired and had given up months ago.

Chapter 14: Crazy Making

"Daring to set boundaries is about having the courage to love ourselves even when we risk disappointing others." Brené Brown

Methamphetamine changes the brain. It uses all the "feel good" chemicals the brain can possibly produce, all at once. A single use leaves a person emotionally frazzled, completely unable to reason or feel any sense of pleasure for a period of weeks to months. Some research suggests that the brain needs 12 months to return to 50% of its normal dopamine production. The only way to feel happy again is to wait it out or to use more meth.

Three weeks after Kurt's relapse we were scheduled to go on a surf trip to Sinaloa, Mexico. Thirty days had gone by and he appeared to be clean. But he was moody and often silently brooding in anger. We were scheduled to surf a private wave. The cartels kept people from surfing this wave unless they were part of our paying group. But the trip was awful. There were no waves. On the two days the swell picked up slightly it was obvious the sand bars at the point break hadn't properly formed that season, making the wave a sloppy mushburger. Kurt stayed in the boat most days while I paddled out with the other men on our trip. In the evening I would do yoga on the beach in front of the surf camp. Several of the men started joining me. The single ones always looked a little differently at me. Or maybe I was looking a little differently at them. But I had to get straight back to our air-conditioned bungalow immediately following my workout, to check on Kurt's latest mood. I missed being chased by guys, guys who didn't use meth and sulk around all day. It would be a few months before I found out that Kurt had gone on a bender just days before our trip, once again stripping himself of any serotonin and dopamine which might have been there before.

Originally I had agreed to give Kurt thirty days. Six months later, the drug had claimed a deeper hold on him than ever before. I wanted to believe him each time he expressed remorse. Sometimes, he would go for a month between episodes. Other times, just a few days would go by before he disappeared for a couple of nights and returned a crazed animal. I could see it in his eyes: a madness that terrified me. Like a rabid dog, he was unpredictable and intensely angry. The smallest thing would send him into a fit of rage, ranting about something I had done horribly or how I had no right to judge him, since he was financially supporting me. Some demon had hijacked his brain and spoke through his mouth. The man I loved was MIA.

He would be sorry, so sorry. He hated himself after each episode. He asked for my help and my support. We went to work and attended group meetings. He got a new sponsor. We went to counseling together. We'd have a great surf session or a beautiful dinner out and everything would feel good again. I remembered how it used to be when we were in love and focused on our spiritual growth.
Then, a switch would flip and the cycle would repeat. He'd go missing. I'd go crazy. He'd come home a wreck, saying he was going to try harder and this time he really meant it. And everything within me would want to believe him.

Finally, I insisted he go to inpatient treatment or else I was leaving him. He refused. He swore he didn't need it. He agreed to go to an outpatient treatment program for three hours per day, five days per week. I hoped the compromise would work. Three weeks later, he disappeared for another four days. He came home with sores all over his body.

One again, I told him it was inpatient treatment or else I was

leaving. I announced that I would get a roommate so he could
be free of paying rent while in treatment. But he would have
none of it.

He agreed to go to sober living, where he would spend his
nights. But he would still leave during the day to go to work.
Just two days into his stay at sober living, I came home from
work to find him watching movies on the couch.

"What are you doing?" I asked. "You don't live here
anymore."
"I don't have to be back until 10:00 pm. I'm already done with
work for the day. There are too many guys at the sober living.
I just need to unwind a bit."

"Kurt, it doesn't work that way. You have to be committed.
And I need my space from you. You are unpredictable."

"That's insane. I pay all the rent so you can live here! I'm
allowed in my own house!" His face reddened.

"I offered to get a roommate so you don't have to pay the rent.
You can't be here." I calmly held my ground.

"Our relationship is falling apart. I don't want to be away
from you. We need to be together so we can work this out."
He was clearly sampling different arguments to find which
might work.

"We can't work anything out until your brain detoxes! I don't
want to be around you like this. Your thinking is totally insane
right now!" I wasn't starting to lose control of my anger too.

"I'm insane?" He got really mad. "You're the one putting
rules on me like I'm a child, and you are financially dependent
on me!"

For the rest of the week, he continued to lay for hours on the couch in front of the TV. I stayed extra hours at work. A week later, he was using again. The sober living kicked him out.

This time, he agreed that he needed more supervision. He enrolled in a treatment program with more supervision, but from which he could still leave during the workday. Once again, I said I would get a roommate. He said not to worry about it, that he wanted to be a provider. He would leave me alone at home but continue to pay rent because "It's what a husband does." My eyes filled with tears. He didn't want to be an addict. He wanted to get better.

This program seemed to be working. He invited me to attend open 12 step meetings with him at the group home. He got permission to take me snowboarding for the weekend. He told me his brain seemed to be clearing, that a fog was lifting. I briefly glimpsed my husband behind all the haze.
A few weeks into the treatment program, I found him back at our house, poking around on the computer.

"What are you doing here?"

"Laundry."

"No, you can't be here."

"You don't set the rules, Natasha! I pay the rent!" He plopped down on the couch and turned on the TV.
"If you have free time, go do something to make yourself healthier. Go to the gym, read a recovery book, take a yoga class. Fuck, just go sit in nature and meditate. The TV is just a waste of time you could be using to get better! You can't afford to sit around wasting time!"

"I work hard, I'm tired and I'm going to fucking rest while I do fucking laundry!"

I grabbed the remote and threw him a book I had just finished on meditation techniques.

"Try this! Or call your sponsor or go be of service or go surf or watch a fucking documentary that won't melt your brain! You're not committed, you're not humble. It doesn't work like this!"

"Oh, and you're so perfect! You have a fucking eating disorder and I pay your bills."

I snatched my purse and stormed out the door. Immediately, my phone lit up, Kurt texting that I was ungrateful and arrogant and that I should go to Al-Anon.

Al-Anon is a program for friends and family of alcoholics and addicts. Kurt thought it might make me less judgmental. Was I judgmental? Was I crazy for thinking he shouldn't be in his own home? Was I being insensitive? After all, he had never hit me or stolen from me. I knew there was a good guy under all that malice. I just didn't know if or when he was coming back. Maybe I was the crazy one, then? So I went to Al-Anon.

Detachment is neither kind nor unkind. It does not imply judgment of the person or situation from which we are detaching. It is simply a means of separating ourselves from the adverse effect of another person's choices.

The detachment flyer, as it is called, is a two-page document containing some of the core teachings of Al-Anon. These were some of the first words I heard, seated in a circle, on a hard metal folding chair on a Tuesday evening at the rec center. The people around me looked just as miserable as I was. A couple of people were smiling, but everyone else mostly glared at them as if to say, "Don't bring that phony ass crap in here, this is where the real shit lives." I had visited plenty of church basement rooms, redolent of cheap coffee and powdered creamer. But the people in these chairs had no facade. They truly knew hell, and they wanted salvation. This was the first public gathering which mentioned God and held group prayer in which I had ever felt comfortable enough to be honest about everything I felt.

The concept of detachment was earth-shaking for me. It meant that I didn't need to get involved in the drama of being married to an active addict. I had been attending Al-Anon for about six months before I finally understood the concept of "detachment with love", or, at least, understood it well enough to move out on my own.

In Al-Anon, we learn not to prevent a crisis if it is in the natural course of events.

Really, I don't have to rush in to save the day?

I revealed to my Al-Anon group that I was thinking of leaving my "qualifier". Qualifier was the euphemism we used to describe the addicts or alcoholics in our lives, those who drove us to attend 12-step meetings of our own, to share our common experiences of strength and hope as it related to living with such people. The meetings didn't allow "cross-talk", which meant we were not allowed to comment on another person's sharing. We could word-vomit whatever we wanted, and there was no criticism or judgment or even advice-giving. The only response you might get from those in the metal folding chairs around you was "keep coming back."

I had been coming back for almost six months, faithfully, two meetings per week. I joined the service committee and even signed up to lead meetings. I found a sponsor and met with her weekly for coffee. I did the homework she assigned. I read the Big Book. I prayed the prayers I found listed therein. I worked the 12 steps, admitting I was powerless over another person's addiction and that my life had become unmanageable, and so on, until I completed the entire program. And I kept coming back. They say, "It works if you work it, and you're worth it, so work it." Those words stuck. I wanted to believe I was worth it. On that particular night, the idea of "I'm worth it" was starting to become more than an idea. I was starting to believe it.

"Hi, I'm Natasha." I begin my share.

"Hi Natasha," the group responded in unison.

"Welcome to the newcomers, I started with the typical introduction. "Tonight I'm exhausted, mentally, physically, and spiritually." I launched into my allotted three minutes of sharing time per meeting.

"You guys, I feel like I'm living with a pissed-off 10-year-old trapped in a very large man's body. It's such a mind game, because I'm looking at the face of the man I am in love with, but the words coming out of his mouth and his body language belong to a monster. Sometimes I believe his venomous words because I don't know if I'm talking to Doctor Jekyll or Mister Hyde. He knows me so well; he knows just what to say to hurt me the most. There are a lot of emotions going on, and I just get so confused. I don't know. I love him. I know that. But I feel like the life is being sucked from me. I feel so small, weak, and fragile. I'm scared...scared there will be nothing left of me if I don't get out. I want to get off this roller coaster. I know I hold the emergency stop switch, and I'm wondering if it's time to flip it. I guess that's it. Thanks for letting me share."

I was leading the meeting that night, so after we recited the Serenity Prayer I headed for the coffee station to set up for post-meeting chitchat. I looked up from arranging cookies and saw three women in their sixties making a beeline for me. Alice gave me a hug and thanked me for my honest share. Linda said she always learned something every time I shared, and also thanked me. Then, their eyes grew serious, as Janet warned me,

"Natasha, if you are going to leave him, and we won't tell you if you should or shouldn't, but if you feel scared, in my experience it will only get worse, so if you are going to leave him, do it when he is at work. Don't tell him your plans; just pack your things and leave. The moment you leave is the moment you are in the most danger."

I fought tears. I wanted to continue the conversation but it was all too overwhelming.

Getting into my car after the meeting, I felt the roller coaster startup. Had I really used the word "scared"? I wasn't scared, maybe just a little *unsure*. Kurt had never hurt me. He would never hurt me. No, I wasn't scared. I didn't need to slip away under the cover of darkness. Kurt and I would have an adult conversation, communicate about what was and wasn't working, and simply take some time apart to sort things out. No big deal.

It had been a few months since Kurt's latest failed treatment program. He was now living back at home with me. Since I had failed to kick him out I kept contemplating the idea of getting my own place to live but money stood in my way. Eighteen months earlier I had opened a yoga studio with Kurt's support. Since that time, four more studios had opened in the same neighborhood. Mine was built on love and a shoestring budget. The others were built with wealthy investors and corporate backers. My self-esteem didn't allow me to ask for a fair price for my classes. I was bringing in only a few hundred dollars profit weekly, despite sixty-hour work weeks. Paying rent and keeping my yoga studio seemed mutually exclusive. Still not convinced that ending my relationship with Kurt was the best option, I turned to my parents for some advice.

They just didn't get it. It wasn't their fault. In their safe little world, my parents didn't know any other people addicted to drugs, nor for that matter did they know any gay people, non-Christian people, or Democrats. Those kinds of people didn't attend their church or homeschool their children, so my parents didn't know them. My parents hated the idea of me leaving the man with whom I had formed a sacred union before God. Or maybe they hated the thought of what their church friends would think about the fact that I had been divorced, twice. Drug use was not a reason to leave. No matter how much I tried to explain the mental games Kurt played with me, my parents didn't get it. I asked them to attend Al-Anon, so maybe they could understand how addicts think and behave. They didn't. It hurt my dad to know that Kurt was "hurting my feelings with his words," so he called Kurt and told him to be nice to me, *because that would do the trick.*

After several unsuccessful attempts at kicking Kurt out, I knew I needed either to accept that he would continue to use crystal meth--and I would continue to watch him sit on the couch watching surf movies, not getting treatment, being the victim of his unpredictable anger--or I would have to get a place of my own. I was petrified. There was no way I had enough income to rent a place of my own. I really didn't even make enough to pay for food and a cell phone. We were at an impasse. Kurt's ego refused to cede control, and I refused to do what it would take to escape a bad situation.

A lot of good friends supported me during this time, listening to my endless drama. One of the reasons I loved my friend Silvia was that she always said what needed to be said, without sugarcoating anything. On a power walk through Balboa Park, Silvia explained to me that I needed to act in my own best interests, regardless of money. The money would work itself out.

"I don't have any other options, Silvia. You aren't hearing me. I can't move out. I simply don't have the money."

We approached the footbridge over the 163 freeway. She stopped and looked into my eyes. She said something only Silvia could get away with saying:

"That's so white trash Natasha. That's battered woman thinking. You are way too educated to live like that. There is always a way, but you are not willing to be humble enough to find it. "

Of course, she was right. I could have asked a friend to let me crash on the couch. I could have packed up and gone home to my parents. I had options, but I wasn't willing to do whatever it would take to get healthy. Not yet. In just a few short weeks, her words would ring inescapably true.

In addition to attending Al-Anon, I began working with a therapist. During one session, I described my terror at watching my savings dwindle, little by little. I told the therapist that I probably had enough to survive for six months on my own. After that, I would not be able to pay rent or buy food. The therapist regarded me for a moment, then asked me the simplest question.

"What happens if you can't pay your rent?"

"I could borrow money from my parents, but eventually I'd have to figure something else out."

"And what happens at that point?" he continued.

"I'd have to close the yoga studio. I'd feel like a miserable failure."

"Ok, so then what comes next?" He wouldn't stop asking the same stupid question.

"Well, I'm not going back to corporate America, and I'm not moving to the ghetto with a bunch of roommates to wait tables. I can't do that to myself."

"So then what?" He was making me think about it like a chess game.

"I guess I'd probably get rid of all my stuff and join the Peace Corps. I've always thought that would be cool."

"That would be AWESOME!" A big smile lit up his face. The smile spread to my face as well.

"Natasha, the universe is like a river and you are floating in the river. The flow of the universe is toward truth and light and joy. All you have to do is stop clinging to rocks. Release your resistance, and just let yourself be carried away. You might get bounced around a bit, but you are always going in the right direction."

The water analogy rocked my world, and I bought into every word of it. The universe is on my side? It was completely different from the it's-all-gonna-burn, sinful nature worldview I was raised on. It resonated in my soul. He then paraphrased what I would later learn was Louise Hay:

"You've never made a wrong decision in your life. In fact, you can't make a wrong decision. You've always done the right thing in the moment you did it, based upon the amount of enlightenment you carried at that time. You have always done your best, and your best is always good enough. By moving toward what makes you happy, you learn exactly what needs to be learned, in that moment."

It was like a math puzzle had just been solved. The universe was on *my* side. I didn't need to suffer to survive. My desires were good and not evil. If I acted on my desires I would be provided for. Taking care of my own needs *and wants* would only lead me to the happiest of places. It would never lead toward doom and destruction. Doing what was in my best interests, there was no way that I could fail.

Now all that was left was to pack my bags and get out of the house.

I had Kandy's number from some family group texts. Kandy was pseudo-family with my in-laws, not technically related, but had been best friends with my aunt-in-law since childhood. At a family birthday party a few months earlier, she pulled me aside to say that if I ever needed a place to stay, I could have her back room for as long as I needed.

At the time, I all but wrote her off. My ego silently asserted that I would never need to take a handout, especially not from an old fat lady whose most exciting part of the day was the New York Times crossword puzzle.

Now, six weeks after Kandy made her offer at the birthday party, I was finally ready to admit the severity of the situation at home. I took a big bite of humble pie and typed out words in a text I thought I would never type. *I can't stay here anymore. I'm starting to get a little scared. I don't really have anywhere else to go. Were you really serious about your offer? I don't have any money and I won't be able to pay for rent right away.*

In less than a minute, my phone beeped with the response. *I'll have the room ready for you tomorrow. I won't accept any money.* The universe had been on my side all along.

He tore open my suitcase and pulled out fistfuls of neatly folded clothing, flinging them around the living room. In contrast to his screams, the clothes hit the wall in silence. They simply lost speed and slid to the floor in crumpled little piles. I, too, dropped to my knees in slow motion, covering my head, heaving silent sobs. When he had finished tearing through my third and final suitcase, the room looked like a hurricane had struck. Pictures were knocked off the wall, and all of my worldly belongings were strewn everywhere. I was in a ball, on the floor, my back to a corner in the wall. My head was between my knees, my hands over the back of my head. Sobs wracked my body.

"Why are you crying?" he screamed down at me. "You want to go? Fucking go, go now, get the fuck out!"

"This is the shit you want?" He barreled around the house, scooping up armloads of the clothes he had just flung everywhere.

"Take it!" Arms full, he kicked open the back door and hurled my clothing into the dark alleyway, where nosy neighbors had already started to peek out of back doors and windows.

His tirade continued. He screamed that I had better tell him where I was going and, if I was staying with a man, I had better be prepared for the worst. How I would end up homeless, since he had been covering the rent for both of us. How I was such a selfish person for not appreciating his generosity. If I had enough money to be on my own, why hadn't I been helping out with the rent? And how I probably had been lying to him for months and stashing away money, and on and on.

The more he yelled, the more I shrunk into myself. I wanted to disappear, to shrink into such a small ball that I could just disappear. *Maybe this was a bad plan. Maybe I should just stick it out with him a bit longer. Maybe he just needed more time. After all, we are husband and wife.*

I'm not sure exactly what happened next, but something inside me snapped. Perhaps it was an animal instinct for survival. Somewhere, deep in my belly, I knew I had to go through with my plan to leave. Curling up into a ball was not going to work. I got an idea.

I would force him to give me an excuse to leave, one that even my parents would accept. I got to my feet and shut off my tears. I emptied myself of emotion. I stood in the doorway, blocking him from returning from the alley, where he was now loading things into my car. I made myself big. He moved like a pissed off bull and he outweighed me by eighty pounds, but I felt no fear. I moved toward him until our faces were inches apart.

I said, "If you are such a big, strong guy, why don't you hit me? Do it, just smack my face. You know you want to. DO IT!"

He didn't hit me. He was shocked. He backed down. He said I was crazy and that he didn't want to hit me. He was right. I was out of my mind.

The neighbors, filled with drama-lust, helped me gather some things from the garage. And that was it. One neighbor asked if I was okay and said she had just called the police for a domestic disturbance, and would I like her to call them back and say we didn't need them. I felt like...well, I felt like white trash. What was a good, wholesome, midwest farm girl with a master's degree in math, a small business owner, and an elected official on the town council doing in an alley at 11:00 pm with the cops about to show up? White trash, indeed.

I drove away, backseat piled with all of my worldly possessions, heart profoundly empty, possessed by a special type of loneliness that follows only from heartbreak or death. I had failed. If only he had hit me, then he would be "abusive". I wouldn't have to feel so guilty about leaving him.

Chapter 15: The Jetty

I decided to believe that taking care of my own needs *and wants* would only lead me to the happiest of places. SoI drove away from financial safety. It would never lead toward doom and destruction. The universe had woven a map for happiness into my fibers. The map spoke to me through desire. All I had to do was treat myself kindly, no matter how scary it got. I must walk through the darkness, because hope and light and happiness would always find me on the other side, in even greater measure than I could imagine.

After a few weeks with Kandy, I found an apartment across the street from my yoga studio. I wrote a cover letter with my application and prayed the landlady wouldn't request tax documents. The next day, I was approved. Three days later, I moved into a space where I could reclaim my dignity. I had no clue how I would afford it. But for the first time in my life, I was completely willing to fail, trusting that the universe had my back, no matter what.

My first day in my new apartment arrived. Since I had left everything except my clothing and personal items behind when I fled my residence with Kurt, I had nothing with which to stock my unfurnished apartment. My friends had supplied me with dishes and kitchen items. Barbara gave me a patio set that needed refinishing that she had never gotten around to doing. Lauren gave me brand new glasses, still in the box. Bryan gave me some cool candles, and Momma Kandy set me up with two rugs, two bath towels, dish soap, and a roll of toilet paper. But I still needed something to sleep on. Mustering my courage, I emailed Kurt to see if he would mind If I took the futon out of the extra bedroom at our old place together.

October 21st, 7:01 pm
*Natasha, I don't agree with or support your decision to sign a lease
and get your own place. I'm not angry about it. I feel it is going to
cause more problems with us, financial stress for you, distance us
more, less time for fun and vacations but if that is what you want, go
for it! Since I don't believe in or agree with what you're doing, I
choose to "detach with love"* [a phrase he borrowed from al-
anon] *and take care of myself. I will not lend or give you the futon. I
will not buy you a futon or a bed. I will not give you any money
during the time we aren't living together. So please do not ask. I
don't care if it's an emergency you will get zero financial support
from me. I feel this is what is best for you. It kind of sucks not having
your spouse's support on something that is important to you and
that you want doesn't it? However, I will be contributing to the
"Fix Natasha's Implant Fund" which now has $1,000 in it."*

He was okay with me sleeping on the hard floor, but he had
the money to fix my implant because that meant bigger boobs.
He always knew just where to put the knife. He was mad
because he had recently tested me in a therapy session, saying
he might not be able to make rent that month and wanted me
to help him out. I declined sighting the many days of work he
had missed the previous month due to being high or coming
down off of a high.

October 21st, 7:04 pm
*Dear Kurt, I understand. I wish you would reconsider the futon
since I got rid of all my furniture to move in with you originally and
since we got the futon as a gift together I feel it is ours and not just
yours but I won't force the issue. I can figure it out."*

His response felt like more acid in my stomach.

October 21st, 7:08pm
*You are correct you got rid of your furniture to move in with me and
then we got married. The futon is at our house that I have been*

maintaining for the past however long and it will remain here. You're a big girl and you decided not to help me or do what I wanted. Now you get to have a taste of what it feels like. I am positive you will have no problem finding another futon or bed. I'm sure someone will help you. Like I said before please don't ask me for any financial help or help period during the time we aren't living together. You have nothing coming from me. You are on your own.

I didn't write back. Eight minutes later, he wasn't finished with me.

I don't know what you expect me to do. I will be nice but I want some respect. I am not gonna kiss your ass and follow you around like a puppy dog. I have proved myself to you and your family. If you aren't willing to forgive me and move on from it that is totally on you.

And twenty-five minutes later, even though I still hadn't responded, he still hadn't said his piece.

This is SO lame. Please file the (divorce) papers, PLEASE! I am begging you for your own sake. You don't want to be with someone like me. There are way better guys out there. They are everywhere! Guys who will build you a yoga studio who don't care if it succeeds or fails. Guys that just want you to be happy. Guys who will give you the financial freedom to do whatever you want. Guys who, even when their wives leave them, still are saving money to help fix the implant that has been bothering you for a long time. Guys who take you on surf and snowboard trips. And most of all guys who aren't drug addicts. I challenge you to find someone better!!!!!! I know I won't find anyone better than you but I can't deal with your bullshit.

There was nothing to say. I went to bed without responding.

He must have fallen asleep angry because the next email

didn't come through until 7:00 am the next morning.

So are you willing to meet or are you gonna keep on thinking I'm a mind reader and keep playing games with me?

Again, I stayed silent. By noon, he wrote me again.

I don't like how I feel and I don't want to not help you even though you wouldn't have helped me. I want to be a better person and not try to get back at you and make you feel how I did. I am going to take the high road & offer to buy you a futon or help you get one. The money will come out of your breast implant fix fund. I am saving it for you so if you want to use it you can. It's for you, not me. If you find one get it and if you need to use my truck you can.

I didn't write back. But I re-read the email thread several times and refreshed my inbox constantly. Somehow, I was addicted to the feeling of each punch. By noon the next day, some of the dope had drained from Kurt's head, and the man I loved wrote another email.

My sponsor said when my medication starts working it should help with my reactivity. Until I calm down I agree that it isn't good for me to communicate.
Healthy Kurt understands and is very proud of you and what you've done. I don't blame you. I told your mom yesterday that I've never been with anyone so healthy and that I'm angry because I can't manipulate or control you. Angry Kurt isn't in control of his thoughts or emotions right now and is pissed. That is the truth and it is hard to admit because my ego, pride, and character defects are out of control and running my life right now.
Despite my bad behavior which I apologize for, I do really love you and would regret losing you.

He wasn't a bad guy. No, wait, he was an awful, manipulative beast. Or was I a terrible wife? Or maybe we were both monsters, or...! My head spun. No futon was worth that kind of emotional rollercoaster ride. I would figure out something else.

I didn't have the money to buy a bed for myself, so I simply turned it over to faith, refusing to grovel in front of Kurt for what I needed.

I went to the swap meet that afternoon to get a few spoons, light bulbs, and all-purpose cleaner. Walking down the aisles, I saw a beautiful, wall-sized tapestry hanging in a booth. I stopped to admire it. A big tree grew from a rock, with all sorts of animals hiding in its leaves.

"You like it?" asked the man at the booth. "It's called 'The Tree of Life'."

"I love it!" I exclaimed.

"I'll make you a good deal, then."

"No, thanks. I can't afford it. It's not on my shopping list today." I studied it a minute longer, lost in its branches.

"Ma'am," a voice called behind me, "do you want that tapestry?"

I spun to see a very large, older black man standing behind me.

"I do want it, but I don't need it," I said.

"Of course you don't *need* it. Who needs a tapestry?" The man laughed. "Sir," the big black man called to the man working the booth, "package up that Tree of Life for the young lady, please."

"Really, no, it's fine. I have more than I need already," I protested.

"But, young lady, you deserve to have nice things too, not just the things you need. God told me to buy this for you, and that's what I'm going to do, so don't argue. Also, ma'am, I'm a pastor. Would you mind if I prayed for you right now?"

I looked at him. I looked at the man taking down my new piece of art. With one hand, I clutched my heart. With the other, I covered my mouth and nose. Sobs gripped my body. I dropped my plastic bag, full of items plucked from the dollar bin, and practically ran to the big black man who now stood with open arms. I buried my face into his grey pocket T-shirt. He rested one hand on my shoulder and lifted the other above him toward the sky.

I don't remember everything he loudly prayed in the isle of that open-air market. But I know he referenced Esther, a woman from the Bible. As the story goes, Esther had to move away from a place that offered her security, because it was the right thing to do. She was so broke and poor that she had to go forage leftover pieces of wheat in the fields, overlooked by farmworkers. But God was looking out for her, and arranged for the farmworkers to leave so much behind that she couldn't even carry it all home.

That night, I lit the candles Bryan had given me. I unrolled my yoga mat, and three more I had borrowed from the studio, for cushions to sleep on. I stared at my Tree of Life tapestry, now hanging on the wall. It didn't even matter that my butt was starting to go numb from the hard floor, barely softened by the four yoga mats beneath me. I felt safe for the first time in a long time. I felt like a princess in a palace. *I'm going to call this place the Princess Cave.*

Reveling in the glory of providing for myself, I heard a
commotion in the alley behind my house. Someone was
dragging something heavy to the dumpster. I heard metal
scraping the ground. A woman's voice announced, "Just leave
it next to the dumpster. Maybe someone will want it."

I got up and peeked out the window. Standing there, propped
up between the dumpster and my back door, my neighbors
had just left a perfectly good futon, a gleaming white mattress,
and a paper bag full of sheets. Esther had a tapestry on the
wall and a bed to sleep in, too.

My new place was an oasis of dignity and respect. I named
my tiny apartment "The Princes Cave". I had no furniture but
I threw pillows, yoga mats, and bolsters around the rug in the
living room. I took cuttings from my neighbors' house plants
and turned my living room into a zen den with loads of
sunlight and greenery. This was the space in which I would
reclaim myself.

On one of Kurt's sober stints, he felt so badly for his behavior
that he ordered me my very first mid-length board. A 7'10"
egg shape, tinted pink and hand-painted by a legendary
female surfer and artist , shaped the board. She painted a
princess riding a unicorn jumping over a rainbow across the
nose of my board. My "princess board", as I called it, would
be the perfect tool to transition toward riding faster waves. Up
until that point I had only rode a longboard. I had my sights
set on a wave simply called, "The Jetty." Jetty waves almost
always tend to be very competitive. They generally form
hollow tubes as powerful waves are slowed by a man-made
breakwater. Often they are quite easy to access since one can
walk to the end of the jetty and jump off. This also means that
they are generally very well attended and the locals don't
always appreciate new surfers showing up to their waves.
Kurt rarely surfed The Jetty due to the hardcore localism in

the water. This only made me want to do it more.

Upon waking my first morning in the princess cave I brewed myself a mug of coffee, pulled on a thick sweater, and walked down to The Jetty to have a look. I stood beside all the other folded arm guys, silently sipping, taking it in. I watched for technical details of the wave. Where the bigger set broke, where the first section occurred, and where it began to barrel. I watched the technical aspects of the surfers' motions; how they angled their take-offs, the precise location of the drop, how they managed to get around the fastest section. I also closely observed the pecking order; taking mental notes of how to behave.

I spent the next two weeks repeating this morning ritual, talking more and more each day with the guys entering and exiting the water. Then one morning I went down to the beach with the princess board. I was nervous, not because of the waves, which looked a little sloppy that day, but because of the locals. When I arrived at the lineup, a couple of the coffee drinking guys recognized me and nodded at me. It was enough to give me a sliver of confidence. I stayed on the shoulder of the wave, far away from the most critical part. I made sure to stay out of the way of everyone else. I only paddled for waves on which someone had fallen or already kicked out of. I think I got three waves that day, and I ate shit on the drop on at least one of them. It didn't matter. I had surfed where I had been told I didn't belong. Nothing bad happened, no one said I shouldn't be there, no one gave me any dirty looks.

For the next year, I made it a point to surf The Jetty at least three times per week. It took a month before I dared paddle for a wave from the most advanced take-off, and another month before I got my first jetty barrel. Slowly I felt something growing inside me, something I would have called self-esteem if I had any idea what it was at the time.

Chapter 16: Boundaries

Although we were separated, neither of us wanted to file for divorce. I knew that an addict inhabited my husband's body. I knew it was possible for my husband to reclaim himself at any moment because he had done it before. I wanted to believe this was just a bad phase. Everything in me cheered for that moment to arrive. But in the meantime, I needed space from his head games. I believed it would be best for us both if he just worked to stay clean and left me the hell alone. I implemented a 10-day boundary. I would speak to Kurt only if he had 10 days clean. Otherwise, he was too reactive and irrational, arguing like a pissed off teenager.

This boundary sent him into another fury. He couldn't wrap his mind around how I could love him and not want to be around him. The drugs had robbed him of his capacity to see the logic in my reasoning. He sent me a text: *You make me so crazy that suicide seems like my best option*, followed by an emoji with an open mouth and then a gun.

That was not the first time Kurt had expressed how upset with himself he was for not being able to kick his addiction, so upset that he wanted to give up and die. I was 90% certain he was trying to draw me into an argument. Detachment (that is, ignoring him) seemed like the best course of action. But after a few minutes, his message started to worry me. I called one of his friends to see if he would check on Kurt, but I got no response. I texted another friend, again no response!

Was I being a little harsh? I mean, I still loved Kurt, I still wanted to be married to him. Maybe I was driving him insane? No, wait, 10 days is nothing. My sponsor had advised a two-week boundary and my therapist had advised me not to talk to Kurt at all. But what if he hurts himself because of my actions?

The mind games ran wild.

So, I called my Al-Anon sponsor. Her suggestion shocked me.

"Well, Natasha, how do you feel about calling 911?"

"What!? No, that would really cause some drama."

"Well, I'm not going to tell you what to do, but that is what the cops are for. And if anything happened to him, you would never forgive yourself. But you don't want to get involved personally, either..."

We hung up the phone and, within thirty minutes, worry overcame me. I picked up the phone. Hands shaking, I dialed 911.

An hour later, an officer called me back. He said he'd found Kurt alone in his home and that, based on his training, he did indeed perceive Kurt to be a risk to himself. Kurt was handcuffed, dragged out of his home in front of the neighbors, and held for evaluation for 24 hours.

Detachment allows us to let go of the obsession with another person's behavior and to lead happier and more manageable lives.

Not long after the 911 incident, I went back to our shared garage to reclaim a few items still stored there. Having been kicked out of his treatment program for relapsing, Kurt was living back in our old home. When he heard me enter the garage, he came to speak to me. I was not in the mood to discuss anything--and Kurt did not have the required 10 days of sobriety. He grabbed me by the arm and backed me up against the classic car parked in the garage.

"Come on. I know we are over, but let's get it on one last time, right here in the car."

He gripped my wrist tightly, his body weight pressed into me. In our relationship, sex was the first thing to go before his relapse. I longed for it, but sex had stopped after he confessed that, because of my weight, he wasn't attracted to me. Now that I wanted nothing to do with him, he was suddenly attracted to me again. He knew just how to play the game.

"No, I don't want to," I stated, clearly and calmly. He didn't let go. Smiling and laughing, he propositioned me again. I had never turned him down in our entire relationship until that moment. I pushed against him with my hips. Panic coursed through my body when I realized I was overpowered.

"NO. Let me go," I asserted again, this time in a loud voice. A neighbor was walking by the half-opened garage door. All three of us looked up at each other. Kurt dropped my arm and stepped back.

A week later, I stood in the lobby of my workplace with a handful of thumbtacks, hanging a new poster. The front door was wide open. Kurt saw me as he drove by. He pulled over. He still didn't have 10 days' sobriety and continued to violate my request for no contact. I had blocked his number and his emails. I couldn't take the ups and downs and mind-manipulating texts anymore. But Kurt couldn't bear the lack of communication. He entered the yoga studio. My intern was there with me. He asked me to step outside to talk, and I refused. He grabbed my hand, dragging me outside, jabbing tack points into my skin.

"I just wanted to say, I love you so much." He had a gift for me. I don't remember what it was, but it wasn't cheap. His eyes were wet.

"I love you too, but you can't be here." Telling him no made my heart feel as if it was shattering. Standing in front of me was my partner, my lover, my husband, my best friend. His tears revealed his own broken heart. The gift displayed his remorse. Yet I knew better. Just behind those piercing blue eyes lurked the addict, ready to pounce. I couldn't. I couldn't let myself be dragged around any longer.

I went back into the studio, and my 16-year-old intern brought tissues for my tears and the blood on my hand. I tried to explain to her how much love can hurt.

A few days later, a big, dark silhouette blocked the daylight from the open back door of my home. Kurt stood there, holding flowers. My heart sank into my stomach.

"You can't be here," I said. "You have to go."

He walked in anyway. He set down the flowers, starting to cry. I started to cry. We both stood there, crying. He said he just wanted to talk.

"I can't talk to you right now. You don't have enough clean time. You aren't rational. You need to leave."

He closed toward me and wrapped his arms around me. Instinctively, I folded my elbows up and made fists, protecting my heart. He held me tight and began to sob. I sobbed too.

"You can't be here, you need to leave," I said weakly. I started to beat my fists on his barrel chest where my face was buried.

"You can't be here, you need to leave." My words were clear, but my body absorbed the comfort of his warm embrace. He kept crying and saying he loved me. I kept resting my head and pounding my fists on his chest, saying he needed to go. Until, finally, he did.

One week later, Kurt was MIA, getting high again. Did holding my boundaries make him feel like there was nothing left worth fighting for? Had I caused him to relapse? Or was sticking to my guns the best thing I could do to protect myself from an active addict?

Detachment allows us to live happier and more manageable lives...we can still love the person without liking the behavior. I still loved him. I was still *in love* with him.

I wasn't happier. My life didn't seem manageable. But the Kurt I loved wasn't there anymore, and this other guy was making me question my resolve.

Detachment can help us to look at our situation realistically and objectively."

Realistically, the only thing I knew was that I was neither realistic nor objective. I knew I was too far in it to see it. I knew I had to listen to the advice of others.

My therapist (the objective one) urged me to put space between Kurt and myself. She showed me a wheel called the "Cycle of Abuse":

Name-calling → Apologizing, saying he won't do it again → Abusive language → Buying gifts to make up for bad behavior → Physical dominance → Making promises or taking steps to change → Accusing the abused of wrongdoing → Going to church, seeking treatment → Physical abuse

...Loving, then cruel, then back again...

My bones turned to ice when she showed me how the pattern worked and also how it progressed. Kurt had never hit me, but everything else on the sheet of paper she handed to me was spot on.

I began to entertain thoughts of divorce--or at least legal separation--to protect myself and my business. I called my lawyer. He said he wouldn't be surprised if I ended up dead, my body dumped off the pier. He said he had seen the situation a hundred times, and the longer the abused party allowed the abuser to carry on, the more dangerous it became.

"Hi, I'm Natasha."

I was always eager to share at my Al-Anon meeting. It felt good to word-vomit. I started right in.

"I know I need space from my qualifier, but I don't want to give up on him. I want him gone. I want him out of my life. But I want the old version of him back. I feel like a widow. It is like my husband has died and a demon has taken possession of his body. I want him to get help, get better, and come back to me the way I found him three years earlier. He wants to go on dates and continue our relationship like nothing has happened. But he keeps using and refusing to go to in-patient treatment and telling me I'm the one causing all the problems because I'm not putting more effort into our relationship. Am I crazy? Maybe it is time to just let it die. Thanks for letting me share."

After the meeting, a man in his late fifties cornered me.

"I had to say something. I know we can't crosstalk during the meeting, but now that it's over, I just have to say this…"

I nodded to indicate I was open to his words, and he continued.

"…I spent twenty years living with an alcoholic. I practiced detachment with her and went to the meetings and I was miserable. Now that I'm out, I have a new lease on life. I wish I would have had the strength to leave twenty years ago. You are young. You have time to start over. Don't wait."

God, grant me the serenity to accept the things I cannot change, the courage to change the things that I can, and the wisdom to know the difference. This prayer opens and closes every meeting.

I was running on fumes. I was exhausted from my work, exhausted from my marriage, exhausted from all the racing thoughts inside my own head. My mental and physical health were spiraling downward quickly.

Like muscles, control and distrust had been flexed within me for so hard and for so long that they were clamped into position. No matter how I tried to relax, spasms reminded me of those hard-flexed muscles. With extreme focus, I could consciously relax the muscle, but if I forgot to relax, the muscle locked up immediately. Control and fear release only with time and effort.

I had faith that, if I rented my own apartment, I would somehow find the money to pay my bills. But the only "somehow" I knew of was working harder. And work took my mind off the pain in my head. I worked around the clock and had agreed to take on another huge project with a business partner: a yoga festival. I hoped it would be good for my yoga brand and lead to a little extra money. Additionally, I served on the local town council as an executive committee member. And I took on personal training clients for extra income. I started every morning with a private client at 6:30 am. Then I would then teach two yoga classes, spend a few hours on administrative work, organize details for the festival, teach another class and then attend meetings for the town council, Al-Anon and therapy appointments until 9:00 pm. Getting out of bed hurt so much, I wanted to cry each morning.

I knew something had to change. There was no way I could maintain the hours I was working, but there was no way I could work fewer hours and maintain a roof over my head. I hadn't bought a latte or a meal out in six months, and none of my clothes fit. Finally practicing a bit of self-kindness I was beginning to feed myself more and I had gained some weight. But I couldn't afford new clothes. The Princess Cave had everything I needed. But it was a little embarrassing when my brother stayed with me and we had to hang out on pillows on the floor because I didn't have any furniture. Or when my sister-in-law visited and we had to share my one fork. Or when my mom came and was appalled that I swept the carpet with a broom because I didn't have a vacuum. But those things were not a priority. Maintaining a roof over my head, a working cell phone, and putting food on the table was the best I could do.

Watching my savings steadily dwindle, I did what a good, hard-working, terrified-to-fail American does: I worked longer hours, with a greater sense of urgency. I cut from my schedule anything that wasn't 100% necessary for growing my business. That included time for preparing meals, daily grooming, cleaning my apartment or car, friendships, friendly chit chat, and definitely recreation and fun. The amount of productivity I could turn out in a single day was staggering. I spent every second being productive for my business. I saw my best month's income at the yoga studio. I made YouTube videos and blogs, posting them to my website. I was doing all that I could do to grow my social media following. I was sprinting to escape the claws of some monster, but the monster was gaining ground. You can sustain a sprint for only so long.

People were starting to notice my decline, and kept saying things like *You can't take care of anyone else before you take care of yourself.* This sounded logical, but it certainly wasn't what I was taught by my self-sacrificing mother, or by the example I had in Jesus Christ, who died for me.

I was in a state of fight or flight. And I felt miserable, physically and mentally. I was gaining weight quickly now. I had no energy whatsoever. I was moody, getting hot flashes at night, and my entire body ached. I was starving all the time. I couldn't remember appointments or where I put my keys. I didn't have the energy to walk a block, but I had to keep teaching yoga classes. I wasn't getting my period, so I had my hormone levels checked. They measured straight zeroes across the board: estrogen, progesterone, and testosterone, zilch.

Sometimes, the universe speaks to us in feathers. You simply follow the feather, drifting in the wind. Other times, the universe bitch slaps you across the face. I wasn't sure what the universe was telling me, but I was sure I was being bitch slapped, and I better listen up.

Chapter 17: Faith

I collapsed on a Sunday morning. I didn't teach yoga on Sundays. It was my "day off", whatever that meant. It was anything but a day of rest. My iPhone calendar displayed a full day. Morning routine, meet with a personal training client, go to church, staff meeting at the yoga studio, meet with John for an Town Council training, back to the yoga studio to write the newsletter and work the front desk, take yoga class, go to Al-Anon, read personal development and film a YouTube video on what I learned, put electronics away by 9:00 pm.

I lay in bed that particular morning, unable to get myself up. I knew all the things that had to be done, and the thought of the day awaiting me felt like a five hundred pound barbell on my chest. "Get up, Natasha," I said aloud. "Get up, you lazy butt!" This last bit was something my mom used to say when I overslept.

I sat up slowly, feeling sick to my stomach. My futon bed was only a foot or so off the floor. I swung my legs over the edge, and a tear welled up in my eye as my bare feet touched the cold wooden floor. I sat on the edge of my bed, both feet on the ground and my head in my hands. More tears emerged. I reminded myself of "the power of positive thinking" or some other crap I was currently reading. *I can do this, I can do this, I can do this*, I repeated the affirmation. I pushed my hands against the bed, and as I attempted to stand, my legs buckled. They simply said *No, you will not be doing this, not today.* I pitched forward, landing on my hands and knees.

I knelt for a moment on all fours, sobs catching in my throat. I saw stray hairs and smeared dirt on the floor as my mind went blank. I closed my eyes and gave up. My body collapsed the rest of the way into a heaving, snotty blob. I lay there, not thinking, not doing, just crying for an indefinite period, in a pool of my own snot and tears.

I remember eventually finding my phone, drafting a text, and copying the same words to everyone I had an appointment with that day: *I'm so sorry I have to cancel today. I had a small family emergency. I will text you tomorrow to re-schedule. Sorry for the late notice.*

I'm not sure how long I remained, weeping onto the hairy, dirty floor. At some point, I became aware that my mind was in a very dark place. I had traveled into the darkest space of my soul. I was terrified, yet seduced to go deeper. Thoughts of blackness filled my mind, longings for a place of nothingness, thoughts that coaxed me further in the direction of letting go, for good. *What was the point?*

I wallowed at length in the darkest depths that morning. It is hard to describe exactly what happened next. Like a seed, dead and buried in the soil for the entire winter, sending out its first sprout, receiving its first sip of sunlight--seemingly out of nowhere, a tiny droplet of painful light pierced my blackness. A gasp wracked my throat, my eyes shot open, my limp body stiffened. My heart cracked wide open.

My next breath felt different, more painful than ever before. But the pain was mixed with a tonic of hope. I knew at that moment that I had hit my bottom. I knew everything about my life needed to change. I knew the most difficult days of my life were imminent. I knew I would have to make massive changes. I knew nothing about my future would be easy. I knew I could, and in fact would make it back to my feet, and that it would be the hardest thing I had ever done. But I knew that, because I *could*, I must... A tiny splinter of hope had wedged itself under a mountain of despair, just in time to

keep the weight of it all from crushing me. 99.9% of me
wanted to give up. Some divine being gave me just enough
strength to draft one more text message.

I wrote the second text and copied it to three of my closest
girlfriends: *I'm not doing too good today. I would rather be dead
than alive. Can you come to be with me?* I had no plan. I knew
only that today would not be the end. It would be the
beginning.

After I collapsed that morning, something inside me changed.
I was ready to do whatever it would take to fix the mess I was
in. The only problem was that I had no idea how.

I made an appointment with my doctor to get some help.
Somehow, the doc saw right through me when I presented
with symptoms of fatigue, headache, weight gain, and
forgetfulness. He refused to diagnose me. Instead, he
recommended yoga and meditation. *Seriously?* Leaving the
doctor without any pills sucked. But if there was one thing I
had learned, it was that I had gotten myself into a huge mess
by my own ignorance, and I better listen to people who knew
more than me if I was ever going to get out of that mess.
Finding my bottom meant I was willing to try any and every
suggestion offered to me. The doctor had suggested that I
needed to make some lifestyle changes, and I knew he was
right. I just wasn't sure how to make those changes. But, being
the straight A student I always have been, I was hell-bent on
figuring it out.

I found a new counselor, one that my insurance would pay
for. I attend gentle yoga classes. I found a progressive church,
filled with supportive people. I bought about ten books on
relationships and drugs and verbal abuse and codependency
and body image. I learned about manifesting. I learned about
thinking big. I learned about bio-hacking. I learned about

honoring my body signals. I learned anything and everything I could do to become a better, functioning human being. I credit Louise Hay, Abraham Hicks, Tony Robbins, Geneen Roth, David J. Schwartz, and Rob Bell with helping to turn my life around.

I learned that when all seems to be in chaos, stick to the basics. So, I started building discipline to make my bed, drink enough water, wash my dishes, go to the grocery store, meditate for five minutes, work out, text a friend, read a personal development book for thirty minutes, listen to an educational podcast while working out, and more. I knew I needed to find time to take better care of myself. My house was in chaos and my clothes stank. These simple tasks seemed to have slipped away during my time of darkness and depression, so I made myself lean into the discomfort of putting one foot in front of the other.

To a healthy person, it seems obvious that I should be doing these things. But to a person who was once convinced that the body and its desires are pure evil, that the world is out to get them and they must struggle to survive, this was a huge step. Each morning, I made time for stretching, reading something inspirational, deep breathing, and food prep for the day. It was amazing, the ripple effect that this basic morning routine had on my lifestyle. That daily practice took up valuable time, which I didn't have. The more I insisted on taking time for the basics, such as doing laundry, putting away dishes, and writing a gratitude list, the less time I had to do work-related projects. I knew I had to choose, work or health.

I felt unbearably guilty telling my 6:30 am client that I could no longer see her. I really didn't have a reason, except that there was no way I could get up at 5:30 to do my morning routine. As a kid, if I slept late, my mom would yell up the stairs, "Get out of bed you lazy butt!" And I felt like a big lazy butt. But no matter how hard I tried, I simply could not do both a morning routine and a 6:30 am client. One of them had to go. To force myself out of bed before I was rested was an act of violence. I could no longer violate my body in that way. My therapist and Al-Anon and personal development reading all told me it was necessary to care first for myself. The client I had to refuse was one of my bread-and-butter clients, and I had no idea how I would go without the money. But the words of my friend Silvia, who had called me white trash for making poor decisions based on a poverty mentality, still rang in my ears. I refused to do something that wasn't in my best interests out of fear of lack of money.

Little by little, I began to make small decisions to put my basic needs above the needs of my business: rest, personal hygiene, cleanliness in my home, healthy eating, and recreation. It was scary, to be sure. Every minute that I spent cleaning my shower was a minute I wasn't spending marketing my classes. Money came in slower and slower. The business, along with my savings, was declining.

Maybe the most important change I made during this time, definitely the most life-changing change I made, was the decision to surf every day.

Surfing is a mission. You have to load the board on top of the car into the racks, drive to the break, get in your wetsuit, paddle out, catch waves for about an hour, paddle back in, get out of the wetsuit, get dried off, load the board back up, drive home, shower, get back in your clothes, re-do your makeup and hair and then get back to work. The whole process takes at least two and a half hours, and it is much better if you have four hours. On top of that, there is no way to stay in shape for surfing except to surf daily. If you skip more than a day or two, you start to lose your surf strength. Then there is the issue of needing to surf when the conditions, tide, swell, and wind are lined up. That is why surfing is a lifestyle.

My lifestyle was work. There was no room to be a true surfer. The problem was that every time I surfed, I felt good. Actually, it was the only thing that made me feel anything other than depressed. Without surfing, I really didn't want to live. Nothing else even came close to giving me hope. Surfing became the reason to get out of bed, the reason to go through my morning routine, the reason to go to the grocery store, the reason to make money.

In the ocean, there is an understanding. I will never win. I will never conquer the wave. There will always be a swell too big to surf. There is always the possibility of drowning or death. Every time I paddle out I admit my own inferiority. And to admit to it is to make friends with it. The ocean makes me acutely aware of my own insignificance. And even so, she still rewards me with a deep sense of satisfaction in my own existence after each wave ridden. I will never win, and I don't care. The other surfers don't care. The ocean cares least of all. I am welcome anew to join her rhythms each day, even if I have nothing at all to offer.

Although surfing is an individual activity, it is actually very social. Since surfing depends on the weather it takes a certain kind of lifestyle to accommodate that, which takes a certain personality. Surfers became my people. The more I surfed, the more I surfed. I started taking off a whole day each week to hang out at my favorite surf spot, kicking it with my friends between sessions. I started taking afternoons off to surf with my friends at sunset. The more time I spent surfing, the happier I got and the worse my business performed. Even my teaching suffered; I just didn't want to teach those people who were paying me pennies.

After a surf session, I would spend as much time as I wanted chilling out with my surfer friends. The energy was always good at the end of a day of good waves. People laughed and told stories about heavy clean upsets or sick little barrels. We would ride skateboards around and smoke pot. I felt like I was having a second chance at a childhood I'd never been allowed to have. Only this childhood involved adult things, like beers, cars, and loads of male attention. If the evening was pleasant, the waves were good and the sunset was a pretty one, we would all pretty much feel like life couldn't get any better. I was experiencing my very first taste of doing life for life's sake, enjoying the present moment with no agenda for the future. And it tasted amazing! At least, until I allowed anxious thoughts of Monday morning's impending doom to pull me from the present and rob me of my joy.

One night, after one of those epic wave days, we nursed some post-surf beers. I sat with Paul and Rifiel, two of the local surfers who ran the break. It was a Sunday evening, and the dread of Monday morning cast a shadow over the epic day. I suddenly felt icky, tension grabbing my chest, ripping me from the present moment. I opened up a bit to my friends. I told them I was sad, how surfing was the only thing that made me happy. I admitted to them that my yoga studio wasn't making much money and required endless work. I revealed that I was trying to recover my mental and physical health, and how much surfing seemed to be helping.

"I don't want to live a life in which I grab occasional moments of happiness. I want to live a happy life and have my work be an expression of that happiness." I pronounced the American dilemma in my own words. My friend Rifiel picked up on what I was saying.

"You could just go to Costa," Rifiel suggested. "Costa" is how surfers refer to Costa Rica.

"It's cheap there. You could just bail on your studio and go. You could just surf all day," he continued.

Those words…" You could just surf all day" slammed into me like a truck. I got quiet. Paul, who no doubt wanted to marry me if only I would leave my husband, also got quiet. I took a long sip off my cheap beer. I looked out into the warm darkness, repeating, "I could just surf all day." I thought for a few more minutes. I thought about what it might be like to live a life that wasn't a struggle, a life where I woke up each day and did only what I wanted to do, a life lived in the present with no worry about the future or guilt over the past. Paul saw the look in my eyes.

"Oh no," he turned to Rifiel, "What did you just do? You shouldn't have said that!"

The idea was planted in my head to take an extended surf vacation. I couldn't stop obsessing on it. My entire body lit up at the idea. I realized that, at thirty-two years old, I suddenly had been handed a second chance at life. Ever since I was a child, I had wanted to travel and see the world. Within each of my romantic relationships, we dreamed and planned for adventures that we never realized. My responsible preparations for the future were keeping me from the present. A steady paycheck, student loans, a new husband, and opening a yoga studio had kept me in San Diego seven years longer than I had originally planned. Now, at thirty-two, I had created a life for myself. I had friends, solid friends who loved me. I was on the town council. I had stuff. I owned two cars. I was established.

But I was slowly losing things too, money, health, my husband, my business...

When I heard Rifiel say I could just go, all of my cells took note that the opportunity for my long- awaited adventure had returned. If I didn't go this time, I might never be able to go again. But I still had a husband with whom I wanted to reconcile. And I had a business. Both felt like anchors around my neck. The more I learned about taking care of myself, the more the idea took root.

Eventually, the guilt of irresponsibility set in. I wasn't doing what needed to be done to run my business properly. The truth was, I didn't give a shit. I was tired of forcing myself to do things I didn't like doing. The time required and the financial gain just didn't add up. Yet, I felt a sense of responsibility to the yoga community I had created. My guilty conscience wouldn't let me quit that easily. I decided to put myself on a surfing restriction. I only allowed myself to surf as many times per week as I actually attended a yoga class. My teaching was becoming stale and I knew it. I knew I needed to practice more and learn from other teachers to improve my craft. I felt I wasn't providing my students with my best.

Focusing on my yoga practice felt awful. Everything in me wanted to spend time outdoors in the salt water and sun. But there I was, on my mat, feeling sick to my stomach. My practice was making me physically ill. I stretched into places that did not want opening. The yoga sutras teach us to practice non-violence as the number one priority, yet I felt that I was committing an act of violence against myself with each yoga class. I simply didn't want to be there.

If everything flows toward expansion and evolution, then I was swimming upstream. I believed that all of creation was moving forward in a grand evolutionary dance. Yet I felt I was dancing in a different time signature. So something had to change. Everything was coordinated, including my body, in the expansion of the cosmos. I had a role to play, a job to do. I had a dharma. My job was revealing itself through my body

signals. My desires were pre-programmed from the beginning
of time to serve as a road map for how to fulfill my dharma. If
the universe was on my side, then my desires were good and
could be trusted. And for the first time in my life, my desires
were loud and clear. I just wanted to say, "Fuck it all, I'm
going surfing!"

Although "Fuck it all, I'm going surfing," didn't seem to fit
any prescribed path toward happiness that I had ever been
told about, my new manifesto meant trusting that my desires
sprang from entirely unsinful origins. If I didn't want to be
doing the job I was doing, then something needed to change. I
was sure that I shouldn't have to be miserable in order to earn
a living. But old attitudes die hard. I still felt that "work"
always needed to involve some measure of suffering. If there
was any way to run my business, make a modest income and
have a few hours of free time daily plus one full day off per
week, I simply had to find it. I knew I deserved that, at least. I
knew that humans were not meant to work like I was.

A friend set me up for a meeting with a very successful
business coach who was wealthier than god and had an IQ off
the charts. This guy was impossible to get a meeting with and
was doing me a big favor. I will not soon forget what
followed.

We met at an outdoor cafe. I ordered eggs. The businessman
took coffee. Between bites, I told him my business model, the
demographics of my location, the size of my building, and any
other details he asked of me. After ten minutes of his firing
questions and my answering, he set down his coffee. He took
a deep breath, looked sideways, and stared into space for a
moment. He nodded his head a bit, and then looked directly
at me. Decisively, he said,

"Nope, doesn't work. Get out."

The friend who had organized the meeting sat with us. Previously silent, he now interjected to defend me.

"Whoa, Natasha isn't looking to become a millionaire. She just wants to teach yoga, pay her bills, and have time to surf."

The businessman thought for about fifteen seconds more.

"Nope, I'd still get out," he confirmed bluntly.

Emotion overwhelmed me. I was quiet. I recognized a familiar feeling. It was the same feeling I'd experienced when Josh admitted to me that he was still watching porn. The same as when I discovered Kurt's relapse. I was neither angry nor defensive. I felt relieved. It was the ticket out that I hadn't admitted to myself that I wanted.

At that point, the only motivation to continue was the fear of failure, the embarrassment of defeat, and the sense of co-dependence I felt for my students. I knew it would hurt. But the thought of giving up made my heart happy. My decision was made. What was left was to act bravely, to pull the plug.

But I clung to Kurt. There was yet one more gift that I was yet too terrified to give myself: permission to obtain a second divorce and love myself just the same. What happened next would be the greatest gift life would ever give me, in the strangest package yet. I was about to know a new freedom and a new peace.

Chapter 18: Life is Too Short to Give a Fuck

I never knew my paternal grandmother. She died young, of breast cancer, before I was born. My aunt, my father's sister, also developed breast cancer when I was too young to remember much of what was happening. I remember whisperings among the family of a genetic mutation that my father carried, the same as his sister and mother. My siblings and I all had a 50/50 chance of having it as well.

BRCA1 is a genetic mutation. Without the mutation, the human body has certain defense mechanisms against rapid cell growth in the tissues of breasts and ovaries. My grandmother and aunt had a mutation, so they were missing this natural defense. BRCA1 is not a gene that causes cancer, but results in the lack of a defense against it. The research and statistics vary, but it is generally accepted that a woman with the BRCA1 mutation is 65-85% likely to get breast cancer in her lifetime (as opposed to 12% of the general population), and she is 45-55% likely to get ovarian cancer (as opposed to 1.2% of the general population). Angelina Jolie, a famous BRCA1 carrier, chose to have a preventative bilateral prophylactic mastectomy. That is to say, she had her breasts removed before they could kill her.

On the phone, my mom told me my older sister had opted to be tested to see if she carried the mutation. My sister had tested positive. She was pretty upset about it and wasn't talking too much. *What's the big deal?* I thought. *So you have it, knowledge is power, get 'em chopped off and get an upgrade.* My mom recommended I think about being tested as well. I didn't need to think about it. I just went ahead and scheduled an appointment.

A quick jab with a needle and it was all over. In a few days, I would know. Five days later, the nurse wouldn't give me the info on the phone. Instead, she set me up an appointment with an oncologist who was also a breast surgeon. *Oh boy.*

I arrived for my appointment, poised and braced. I was in the middle of everything with Kurt and I had become an expert at wearing my tough girl mask. I was unshakeable. It was no big deal. I went to the appointment hungry, in one of my "beat my body into submission with some stupid low-something diet" phases. I blasted loud, you-can't-mess-with-me ghetto rap in the car on the way to the appointment. My phone pinged while I drove. I looked down to see a paragraph-long text from Kurt. He did not have the ten days clean from using meth I required before speaking to him. The text was something about how self-righteous I was for having this rule, and how my Al-Anon program and my boundary-setting were "fucking our marriage". It was going on a year since his first relapse. and he still couldn't get more than a few days clean at a time. Still, I was hoping against hope that he would pull himself together.

Although I had been living on my own for a few months, I held out hope for restoring my relationship with Kurt. He would go to a treatment program, then relapse and get kicked out. He would go to three meetings a day and then relapse. He would go to a sober living and then relapse and get kicked out. He would move in with a sober roommate and go to outpatient treatment and then relapse and get kicked out. I wanted to wait it out. He wanted to get clean. He hated himself for using. I loved him. I was *in love* with him. But I was slowly dying inside. He was getting worse, not better. I clung to less and less.

Every day, I prayed for him. We shared brief moments of reprieve in which he collected a few weeks of sobriety and restored his rational brain. We laughed or engaged in a productive therapy session or make-up sex. One time, he even picked me up in a limo, wearing a suit from the '90s, holding a dozen red roses. I'd let him back in and a few days later he would disappear, eventually to resurface after going MIA. He returned each time a little meaner than the time before. He didn't want to be using it, but he wouldn't stop. He refused to go to a long term inpatient program because he didn't want to lose his job or his apartment. He constantly bought me gifts, sent me flowers, wrote me postcards, and then relapsed. Then he'd send me name-calling texts, blaming me for his using and refusing more treatment. Admittedly, I didn't always handle these nasty bouts very well.

Bobbing my head to the ghetto rap, I deleted the text before his words could sting too much. I wrote him back, *Call you later when you are ready to have a non-abusive adult conversation. On my way to find out how soon the cancer monster is coming for me, can't talk now.*

I parked my car and strode confidently to the elevator. I punched in the floor number I had been given for the appointment. The lights in the office building were too bright, the tiles too white and too shiny, the halls too echoey. I wore wedge heels with my designer yoga pants, trying to look put together. The heels clicked loudly as I searched for the clinic door. *Stupid shoes.* I noticed a sick feeling in the pit of my stomach. *I should have brought something to eat.* I was shown to a little room with two chairs and an examination table. I sat on the crinkly paper on the table and scrolled through Instagram while I waited for the doctor.

A doctor, a resident, and a nurse walked in. The resident and the doctor sat in the chairs, the nurse stood. The room felt cramped. The doctor delivered the news, which did not shake me. The test result had come back positive: I carried the genetic mutation BRCA1, the same mutation that had killed my grandmother and taken my aunt's breasts, and scared the crap out of my sister. I did not blink. I did not move.

"Then I want it all out," I blurted, interrupting the doctor who was carefully choosing her words so as not to scare me.

"Let's do this," I continued with resolve, "chop off my boobs and make me better ones. Take out my ovaries, I don't want babies anyway. That way none of my defective parts ever have the chance to kill me."

My doctor paused. A beautiful woman in her 50's with botoxed skin, wearing stilettos under her white lab coat, this woman was not amused by my brusque bravado. Her tone shifted.

"Natasha, do you have any idea what that even means?"

Her eyes narrowed, and she didn't wait for me to answer. She went on, "We are talking about scraping every bit of tissue from the inside of your breasts--from your underarms to your sternum, you will be disfigured. Then we have to go back in and stretch out what's left with expanders over the course of two or three more surgeries. You will have scars from your armpits to your nipples, but you won't have nipples anymore because we have to take those too. You will wear drains externally, as fluid runs out of the spot where your breasts used to be and pools in plastic bags that you will have to tuck into pockets sewn to the inside of a cardigan. The average woman goes through 4.5 surgeries, and her breasts never look as good as cosmetic implants because there is absolutely no natural breast tissue left to disguise them. Then there are the phantom pains that will haunt you for life as your body tries to make sense of what is missing. And you want your ovaries out, too? You are talking about instant menopause. Your skin will wrinkle and sag, people will guess your age to be ten years older than you are. You will *feel* ten years older because your body will ache with joint pain. Your sleep will suffer and you will have a huge drop in energy because of it. With joint pain, low energy, and poor sleep, you can forget surfing, yoga, and running at the level you currently enjoy, which likely means weight gain, which means more joint pain and more poor sleep, and the nasty cycle gets worse."

"What about hormone replacement?" I stood up to her, still playing tough girl...*I've done my research, darn it!*

"Right, pump your body full of the stuff that causes breast cancer in the first place? Natasha, I'm not trying to tell you what to do. I'm simply saying you are young, you just found out, you need to think this through a little. You mentioned some issues with your marriage. Now is not a good time to make big life decisions. I won't operate on you now, even if you want it. The research shows that women are living just as long with their breasts intact. You just have to stay healthy and do the screenings. Ovarian cancer is a much scarier issue. We don't have good screenings for it and it isn't typically caught until it is very advanced. Your family history presents with issues around age forty-five. I recommend having children as soon as possible, and having your ovaries removed in ten years. In the meantime, try following some of the women on Instagram who've had these preventative procedures. What you want me to do will affect your entire life, as you will see."

I shut my mouth. I blinked several times, expecting tears. They didn't come. *I am too hard for tears.* She said the nurse would go through a few more things with me and she turned to go. I heard her stilettos click on the cold, white tile floor toward the door. She opened the door a crack, then turned around.

"Hey," she smiled for the first time, "Just be happy, do things you love, live your life. Attitude goes a long way in prevention."

I walked down the too-bright hall toward the elevator, wanting badly to cry, but my toughness wouldn't allow me to crack. I pushed the button for the parking ramp. The elevator started to drop. I made a mental list of my options:

1. Remove body parts, not get cancer.
2. Wait and remove body parts once they become cancerous.
3. Fight like hell.

I got back in my car, turned off the ghetto rap. I sat silently within the dark ramp. In my head, I chanted the words of the doctor, *Be happy, live your life, be happy, live your life, be happy, live your life.*

Suddenly I was too worn out to give a fuck about anything anymore. I started the engine, buckled my seatbelt, put the car in reverse but didn't take my foot off the brake. I sat there, thinking. I put the car back into park. I dug my phone out of my purse. I texted Kurt.

I'm done. I'm out. You will have divorce papers by the end of the week.

After hitting send, I tapped the block button next to Kurt's number in my phone. I turned up my ghetto rap, backed out, and drove away, bopping my head.

Chapter 19: Surrender

I had already trusted my gut enough to leave my husband, rent my own apartment, file for divorce, cut back on work, and list my business for sale. I trusted my appetite for dignity, rest, and even for little bits of pleasure. But I still fought my appetite for food. I was terrified that if I actually let my body have what it wanted, I would gain weight. It was my worst nightmare.

The more I read on the subject, the more I began to accept the facts: if I wanted to be healthy, I needed to convince my body that there was enough food. That meant trusting my hunger. Giving in to my hunger was awful. The full power of the primal brain, inside an animal that has been underfed for the last fifteen years, unleashed itself within me. Everything in me screamed for food, for the feeling of fullness, like lungs crying out for oxygen underwater. My body needed to be fed. For the first time, I was going to listen to it. Of course, I had given in to hunger many times before, in binges. But I had always followed by making myself vomit, which only made me hungry again in an hour.

There was a longing in the way I didn't eat. I wanted to be full--full of meaning, value, status. There was never enough. You had to endure if you wanted something. I wanted people to want me. I didn't know I wanted peace. My wanting separated me from what I already had within me. Eating disorders are about forgetting. Having forgotten what I was, I went on a desperate search. And now the search had led me to a place I no longer wanted to be. The longing had to be satiated.

I wanted to be ready to give up the last little bit of control. But it wasn't that easy. I resolved to try it, if only for a day. I decided to throw out all my food rules and try to live by only three new rules; 1) eat if my body was hungry, 2) eat what it was hungry for, and 3) stop only when I was full. If my body was good and the order of nature was on my side, then at least I had to try to trust my body.

The first binge without a purge was the worst. After half a loaf of gluten-free bread and half a jar of almond butter, I felt "sorta" satisfied, but also panicky. I went back for three more slices of bread until I felt definitively "full". I knew I had just eaten enough to actually gain weight. This wasn't just like eating a little dessert and feeling guilty. I really, really was going to gain a pound or two of pure fat from what I just ate. The food felt like poison inside my belly. I wanted to put on a men's XL T-shirt and sweats. I wanted to bury myself in a hole.

"Sit with the discomfort" was something I told my yoga students. I couldn't get it out of my head. That moment was pivotal for me. I remember closing the fridge and crying as I walked to my bedroom and got under the covers, though it was only mid-afternoon. I sobbed hard. I slammed my fist into my pillow. I felt like I wanted to be lower, so I climbed out of bed and laid face down on the bare, wooden floor. A little pool of snot and tears gathered under my cheek, reminding me of the last time I had been in that position. I pushed my face into the grimy floor, trying to get smaller and lower.

You will lose your beauty.

I don't know where the words came from. The voice wasn't audible, but it was from outside me.

You will lose your beauty, and you will gain your soul.

And it wouldn't shut up. Over and over,

You will lose your beauty. And you will gain your soul.

You will lose your beauty. And you will gain your soul.

"NO!" I shouted. "NO! I can't, I won't, don't make me go through this!" I begged and I sobbed, but I knew the voice could not be bargained with. Surrender was my only option.

The second binge without a purge sucked just as much. The seventh and eighth times were no better. But I didn't purge. I let myself eat as much as I wanted, and I had to keep it in. At first, I simply could not get enough food. No matter how much I ate, I didn't feel satisfied. Sometimes I ate enough for four or five meals at a time. Over time, my body recognized how awful it felt to eat that much food at once. Eventually, binges turned into XL portions and frequent meals.

Like a wild animal, hunger was the driving force to move each morning. The first thing I did was to make a huge bowl of oatmeal and a protein shake. Within an hour or less, I was hungry again. I would make a veggie omelet. After teaching my first yoga class, I would be famished and return home for a large salad with lots of olive oil and chicken. By noon I was ready for lunch. It would go on like this all day, eating a full meal, large and healthy, almost every hour. I was committed to listening to my hunger, and I was physically starving.

My weight did indeed change. After several months I gained around 30 pounds. I felt absolutely disgusting. I had to buy new clothes, twice. My thighs chafed when I walked in my bathing suit. I couldn't do many of the yoga poses I easily used to do. I couldn't stand the sight of myself in the mirror. It often provoked tears. I took a whiteboard marker to my bathroom mirror, writing things I loved about myself all over it. I hung a sheet over my full-length mirror, so I didn't have to see. I lived in yoga pants and avoided jeans at all costs. Many times, when I wanted to go out with friends, I would try on everything in my closet and end up in tears, texting my friends to cancel plans. I just couldn't stand to bring my fat self out in public.

I had never been that heavy in my life. Even though I loathed the sight of myself, I clung to some tiny bit of faith that this was indeed the process my body needed in order to heal. After gaining four dress sizes, I still had no energy. I still wasn't getting my period. I was still starving all the time, and my faith was dwindling. This stupid body could not be trusted after all!

Thanksgiving rolled around. I was terrified of being without my family, and now I didn't have my in-laws to celebrate with either. Mustering humility, I asked a girlfriend if I could spend the day with her family. We ate well, we overate, and we ate dessert. After all, it was Thanksgiving. Returning home to the Princess Cave that night, I found the heater turned off. It was cold and lonely after the laughter of my friend's family. My belly felt fatter than ever. Even though I had been feeding myself well for months, I still clung to "safe foods" and never ate things like pumpkin pie and mashed potatoes.

The Voice sounded so much like my own that night that I believed it actually was. *I hate this stupid body! I've been trying to listen to it for a year, and all it is doing is getting fat. I'm not getting healthier, I'm getting FAT. I'm not learning to listen to my hunger, I'm getting FUCKING FAT! FUCK THIS, FUCK ALL OF THIS!*

I put my hair in a ponytail, heading for the bathroom. I lifted the seat and dropped to my knees. I stuck my finger down my throat. I gagged once, twice, three times. But nothing happened. Nothing came up. I found my toothbrush and stuck the handle down my throat. I coughed and it hurt my throat, but still nothing. I was such a fat, miserable failure that I couldn't even make myself vomit anymore. I crumpled to the bathroom floor in tears. I had never hated my idiotic body so much in my life.

And the worst thought of all was that Kurt was probably telling all his friends he dodged a bullet referring to my weight gain. I still missed him like crazy. The divorce was in process but a mandatory six-month waiting period kept it from being official. I prayed every day for a miracle, that he would wake up and snap out of the trance.

Change happens when the discomfort of the present moment outweighs the uncertainty of the future. My life had become difficult enough to step out into the ambiguity.

I was miserable. I was heavier than I had ever been, constantly feeling ill and nearly completely out of money, I was heartbroken. I was trusting the universe to provide, and I was feeling a nudge for even more surrender. I hadn't given up control completely, I was still fighting daily to keep an income source flowing.

I was just about to finish up a major yoga event which would put a little money in my pocket. I had a choice to make. Reinvest the money into my yoga studio or make a change.

I wasn't born a surfer, but the ocean flows through my body. All of life was conspiring to return me to my salty home. There was really just one thing in my life making me happy. Surfing. Of course, I had no idea how surfing would pay the bills. But it didn't matter. My desires could be trusted and I

wanted to go surfing. I needed to go surfing. I wasn't willing
to force my body back into exhaustion mode just to survive. It
felt like the first time in my life that I actually knew what I
wanted and I wasn't too paralyzed by the guilt of what I
should do to go after it. I understood that healing my
relationship with food meant trusting my intuition fully. It
meant being kind to myself. It meant setting my heart free to
lead the way.

My friend Rifiel had given me the idea that I could just leave
and travel and surf. The idea would not leave my mind. I
stayed up late, researching where I might like to go and the
cheapest places, where I could stretch my money the farthest.
I researched Indonesia, Panama, and Mexico. At first, it was
just a silly idea. I had lived in San Diego for almost ten years. I
had friends, responsibilities, and stuff. I was comfortable.

The yoga festival put a little chunk of money in my pocket,
maybe enough to pay my bills for a few months if I lived
cheaply abroad. Some deeply hidden, rebellious part of me
longed to say "screw it, I'm outta here!" and to leave on a new
adventure that would last for the rest of my life - screw being
skinny, screw being in love, screw building my career, screw
doing the right thing with my life. I just want to eat and surf
and travel and fuck whoever I want, whenever I want, as
much as I want. I want to do what I want to do for the first
time ever. Is that so bad? Am I such an awful human for
admitting that I want something? That I want sex and
adventure and a full belly? Am I a sinner for saying that?
Then label me a sinner, because I don't fucking care anymore!

But my conditioned side reminded me that this was crazy.
You don't just leave your life and travel indefinitely without a
financial plan! Do you? No, no, no, I would come up with a
plan. I would leave for just a little while and return to my life
when I was a bit more rested. Yes, that was the responsible

thing to do.

I found a boutique resort in Mexico willing to board me in exchange for playing hostess. There was surfing right out front and two meals a day were included. My choice was made. I told everyone, including myself, that I was going away for just over three months--one hundred days. I made arrangements to be able to return to my life when I was done. I subleased my apartment and locked up my garage. My yoga studio was still running, so I put a manager in charge and told her the position was temporary, that I would be back in 100 days.

PART II - Surf

Chapter 20: Leaving

I don't remember how I told Sean that I wanted to be free to sleep with other men while I traveled, but I do remember that I was standing in his kitchen when I did it, and that saying the words felt like passing kidney stones. In every previous relationship, I wanted out long before I let myself out. I always looked for something that my partner did wrong to give myself permission to leave. Sean came into my life shortly after I filed for divorce. He was wonderful, an engineer with an Ivy League education, a homeowner, a hip-hop DJ, a feminist, and a dedicated surfer. It never occurred to me that a man could be perfectly good, yet I would still have different desires for my life. Telling him I wanted to be single felt like I was telling him he wasn't good enough for me, which felt harsh. And it took a massive leap of faith to speak my desires out loud. Not only was I beginning to have faith that my desires were healthy, but I was starting to be able to admit to having them. This process, it turned out, was just beginning because I still wasn't strong enough to tell Sean the whole truth. I hadn't even told myself the whole truth. Sean asked me for how long I thought I would be gone. I told him the same lie I was telling myself: 100 days. He seemed like the ideal man for me to live happily ever after with. He was nothing but supportive of my need to take a surf trip. He himself was well-traveled and understood the value of what I was doing. He promised to visit me while I was away. He even agreed to help me make the drive down to Mexico.

I *wanted to want* to be gone for only one hundred days, and then return to my beloved little ocean side town, my amazing yoga students, my 1971 cherry red convertible, my boyfriend, and my Princess Cave. But I knew I was fooling myself. I found a manager willing to run the yoga studio while I was gone. I found a friend to sublease my apartment. I really liked many things about my Southern California life, my Princess Cave, and my classic car and camping gear and snowboard equipment and designer heels and artwork and boxes of books, all stored in my garage. *Yes, I would be back in one hundred days, right?* But I knew in my heart the mistress of adventure is a jealous one. "You can't have this if you want all that and you certainly can't have me." She whispered in my ear.

Saying goodbye to my Al-Anon friends was the easiest, because the only thing we Al-Anoners know how to do is support each other. Leaving my church was harder. Leaving the town council gave me incredible guilt. I felt like I was leaving them hanging, like I had let down my fellow Obecians. Saying goodbye to my yoga community was the most guilt-inducing of all. No one knew I planned to sell the studio as soon as I had a buyer. I told everyone I'd be back in three months, but the tears I cried at the end of the last class I taught revealed what I knew in my heart: this was goodbye.

The hardest was leaving the guys with whom I had wasted so much enjoyable time, watching waves with folded arms and swapping stories after epic days of surfing. Paul helped me pack my truck and hugged me goodbye, fighting back his own tears. Richy warned me I would end up dead in a Mexican ditch and told me not to go. Chad, who had done nothing but support me for our entire friendship, said he was jealous and told me to enjoy every moment. Rifiel laughed and claimed it wasn't his fault.

Leaving Kurt was the easy part. He still hurt me every day in my thoughts. His manipulative words still hung in the air I breathed, even though we hadn't talked in a few months. I needed to escape. As long as I continued to live a life that looked anything like our old life together, I would not be free of this pain. Everything had to change. And I knew it.

The hotel I was to work for informed me that I'd need a car. They suggested I drive down. I was nervous but excited. My plan was to drive for three days through Arizona and northern Mexico. The first part of the drive was all on well-maintained freeways. After three days, I was to meet Sean in Guadalajara, where he and I would drive together for five days, surfing a few locations along the way.

I bought a 15-year-old Honda CRV, a small SUV with decent ground clearance, all-wheel drive, and room for my gear. I would have preferred something newer but adventure being what it is, my budget was going to throw me some curve balls including a used vehicle with high miles.

Day 1

The fateful day arrived. I had a playlist prepared for the occasion. I handed over the keys for my apartment to my subletter. I tugged on the straps securing my three surfboards to the roof of my truck. I popped a bottle of water into the cup holder. Paul took a photo for me, and away I went.

I hit the gas as I turned onto I-8 East, headed to Arizona. My plan was to spend the night in a border town, then drive two hard days to the inland city of Guadalajara, Mexico, where I would meet Sean. He would assist me with the rest of the drive to the resort town of Troncones, Mexico. I was terrified of the two days of solo driving, south of the border. Anyone who hadn't done the drive warned me not to do it. Anyone who had done it told me it was all nice toll roads, and I would be fine. As I merged onto the 96 East, outside the San Diego city limits, I texted my best friend back home in Michigan.

OMG Kate, I'm doing it!

Adrenaline and good music pumped as I crossed the California border into Arizona. *Here we go, here we go, here we go!* The cruise was set to 80 mph. I hugged the left lane and I felt I could take on the world.

WHAM! SMACK! I screamed, the car lurched left. The rumble strips were deafening. Something black smashed into the driver's side window as I slammed on the breaks. I hit the hazards and pulled off to the side of the road. The traffic flying by felt like it would suck my truck back onto the freeway. I opened the door to have a look. My front driver's side tire was completely shredded. A six-inch piece of rubber running the entire circumference of the tire had come completely loose and must have hit the front bumper as it flew off. The bumper was hanging by a thread.

I got back in the car. I started to cry. *This was a sign I shouldn't be doing this. God was punishing me.* Guilt overwhelmed me. Suddenly I was starving. I reached for my bag of snacks and tore open the first package I could find. I sat there, munching salted almonds, numbing the fear. The Voice started in on me,

What now? What have you gotten yourself into? What have you done? Why did you give up such a wonderful life? What were you seriously expecting? You are crazy. You are stupid. You are ignorant, You are ungrateful!

I ran through my options. The first thought was to turn around, go back to safety, admit defeat. I would ask a friend if I could stay with her. I would get a waitressing job. Or maybe I would go back to Michigan and live with my parents. I picked up my phone to call Sean for advice...*no I don't need him.* I put the phone down. I picked it back up to call my Mom, *No way. I definitely don't need her.* I put the phone back down. More traffic whizzed by and my truck was shaking. I picked my phone up this time to call AAA to renew my membership. I Googled the number and hit send. I was on my own now. I could figure this out. *Time to put your big girl panties on, Natasha!* I would tell no one until after I had already found a solution myself. I could do this on my own and I was going to prove it!

One tow, four new tires, ten zip ties in the bumper, and three hours later, I was back on the road. I uploaded the first photo of my trip to Instagram: my truck on a flatbed wrecker, with the caption, "Nothing I can't handle!" If I had known how minor this was compared to what I would later face, I may have given more serious thought to The Voice when it urged me to admit defeat. I found a truck stop still on the American side of the border. It would be the first and last time I would ever sleep in a truck stop parking lot.

Day 2

I was ten minutes over the Mexican-American border. I knew from my research that I would need to buy an immigration sticker for my car. I tried to read the signs to find the kiosk, but nothing made sense. I pulled over at an official-looking government building and asked the guy trying to sell me bracelets and straw hats for Immigration Services. He started speaking very rapidly through his toothless grin. I understood nothing. I used my best Spanish to ask him to speak slower, but it didn't help. But he was pointing toward a building in the same parking lot, so I locked my car and went in the direction his finger indicated.

I looked back over my shoulder as I walked away. My whole

life was in that truck. There was no way to really lock the surfboards strapped to the top. Feeling like a sitting duck, I walked into the building, my car out of sight. After half an hour of hassle, I figured out where to buy the immigration sticker and paid a hefty deposit on my credit card, promising I would take the car out of Mexico within 180 days. Though it was much longer than the 100 days I planned to stay, somehow I knew I would not be getting my deposit back.

Within a few miles of being back on the road, I encountered the first toll booth. I saw the fee listed in pesos, did a quick conversion in my head, and handed the attendant three US dollars. She shook her head and handed the money back to me.

"You don't take dollars?" I was surprised because in all my travels in Baja Mexico, you could always pay the tolls in either currency. She responded with something about pesos. I tried to argue, but she didn't speak any English. In Baja, I hadn't had a problem getting by on the few Spanish words I knew; most people I encountered spoke some English.

You stupid idiot, The Voice mocked, *This isn't Baja, you don't know SHIT! One year of Spanish classes over a decade and a half earlier, what were you thinking? Look what you got yourself into!*

Luckily, I had a few pesos from my last trip to Baja, so I handed over all the Mexican money I had. She handed me back the equivalent of about 1 US dollar. I was going to need to find a currency exchange, and fast. Within a few miles, I located a store with signage that seemed to indicate they would exchange money. I locked the car and once again worried about the surfboards on top as I made my way inside. A girl of about fourteen was working the counter. I told her I wanted to exchange money. She had no idea what I said. I realized I had no idea how to ask her in Spanish. I also realized my translator app would not work without a wifi connection. After about twenty minutes of sign language and pure frustration, I walked away with enough pesos to get me through the day. I knew I paid way too much for them.

As I got back in my car, a realization came over me: I was in way over my head. Somehow, I had thought my year of eighth grade Spanish Language and my limited trips to Baja to surf prepared and qualified me for an international move to the developing world. I was ignorant, not brave, and at that moment I became aware of it. I took three deep breaths and made up my mind to become brave. I blasted my music and spun out as I pulled away.

I drove until dusk that night with an iron grip on the wheel. I found a decent hotel in a medium-sized city and made sure to send WhatsApp messages to my mom and Sean, assuring them I had made it safely behind a locked door before dark. Sean requested that I send him a pin, showing exactly where I was. I did. I slept great and woke early, ready for my second, and last, day of solo driving in Mexico.

Day 3

The day started with an ice-cold beet juice in a plastic bag with a straw, which I bought from a child selling juices at a speed bump in the road. It was so good, so fresh, so cold! Later I stopped at a roadside stand for tacos. I noticed a group of men eating a fish with the head and tail still on. I had never before seen a fish served whole. I pulled out my phone to take a video. The guys thought I was really quite a sight, the only white person for miles in any direction. They laughed and indicated I should try the fish. I didn't grow up with seafood and had always hated the taste. But fuck it, this was an adventure, Buen Provecho! I reached my dirty hand right into the body of the whole fish like I saw the men doing. I plucked out a piece of the flesh. It was crispy and greasy and salty...and delicious!

My plan was to make it that evening before dark to Guadalajara, where I would get a hotel room and wait to meet Sean when his flight arrived the next day. I looked at the mileage and time I was averaging, and calculated that I would be cutting it close to arrive and find accommodations before dark. I stepped on the gas pedal a little harder. As I glanced down at the speedometer, my heart dropped into my belly and my breath caught in my throat. The check engine light had come on. OH SHIT! I was in the middle of nowhere. I hadn't seen a service station or a town in the last hour and my phone had no coverage. My AAA membership was not going to work here!

You stupid idiot! Why did you buy such a cheap car? Why did you buy a car less than a week before your trip? You are so arrogant! I can't believe your ego! Now you have a lemon on your hands and you are going to be stranded here and at the mercy of the Mexican Cartel! Everyone was right, this was a bad idea! What were you thinking?!

On and on, The Voice belittled.

I pulled the car over and checked the oil. It was fine. I checked the coolant. That was okay, too. I didn't know what else to check. I got back on the road and continued in the same direction, praying for a town to appear soon. I listened to the engine, and it did seem a little funny. It felt like I had less power as I went uphill or tried to accelerate quickly...or was I just making that up? I stopped at the first business I saw, a small shop of the type common in Mexico, filled with beer, beverages, cookies, and chips. I asked for a mechanic. They said the name of a town. I asked, "Que lejos?" They said one hour, inland, out of my way.

It was actually over ninety minutes before I found the town, and another three stops, with frustrating attempts at communication and a prayer each time that the engine would start back up. Eventually, I arrived at a mechanic shop. For some reason, I said a prayer: *Dear God, please give me a female mechanic.* I was so nervous, and somehow I felt a woman might understand more than a man what I was going through. But I wasn't sure if they even *had* female mechanics in Mexico.

As I walked in the shop, I was greeted by a woman in bright red lipstick, high heeled wedge shoes, skin-tight skinny jeans, a classic mechanic's greasy navy button-down, and a wrench in her front jeans pocket. I took a deep breath. I was going to be okay.

After an hour under the beating sun, struggling to communicate through a mixture of sign language and Google Translate, I would understand that it was an oxygen sensor setting off the check engine light. Mexican gasoline was notorious for blowing out O2 sensors, and although I would experience decreased power and fuel economy, I was safe to continue on my way.

The setback cost me four valuable hours, and I knew I wasn't going to make it to my destination before dark. I had built in an extra day of leeway, just in case something like this happened. I enacted my contingency plan, pulling over in the resort town of Mazatlan, where I splurged and stayed at a high rise hotel for the night. I was given a room on the eighth floor. Reluctant to leave my boards strapped to the roof of the car, I locked the smaller ones inside and took the biggest one with me. But when I tried to get my longboard in the elevator, it would not fit. A generous bellhop carried my nine-foot board up eight flights of stairs to my room. As I drew back the curtains, I took in the view of the Pacific Ocean. *Wait a sec!* There was a wave breaking right out front! It was tiny, almost unsurfable, but surfable. I couldn't get a fin in my longboard or wax on it fast enough. I had maybe forty-five minutes before dark. The guests looked at me like I was crazy as I dashed down eight flights of stairs in a bikini, lugging a giant blue surfboard. The first splash of warm salt water felt like heaven. I giggled and laughed as I rode ankle high waves. Finally, I had reached warm Mexican waters!

Day 4

The next morning, I carried my board back down eight flights of stairs. I loaded up my boards, back onto the roof racks. But when I went to tie them down, the entire mount shifted. I checked the bolts. Someone had attempted to loosen them overnight, but was stopped by the locking mechanism. The sickening feeling of violation soured my stomach.

I told the security guard in the parking lot what had happened. He appeared as if he didn't understand. I dug in my toolbox, which I had carefully packed, finding an Allen wrench to secure the racks back in place. *Good heads-up thinking on packing the tools. Proud of you, chica!* Must have been The Voice was in a good mood that morning.

By the time I reached Guadalajara, I was drenched in sweat, despite icy cold AC blasting in the car. My head throbbed and my throat felt like needles. I told myself I was just tired. But when I finally checked into a hotel, I couldn't seem to get to the bathroom fast enough. A thought crossed my mind...how was that beet juice yesterday so cold? The bags of juice were out in the broiling sun. The only explanation was ice. Ice from the side of the road, and tacos from carts and whole fish with the head still on...I hadn't been careful at all. I had been ignorant and arrogant, again. The buzz from the adventure started to wane as I sweated out my arrogance in a dumpy Mexican hotel room.

Change only happens when the pain of the status quo outweighs the fear of the unknown. I considered myself lucky for being too stupid to be afraid. Had I known what I was in for, I would have needed to hit an even darker, deeper bottom before I overcame the fear of packing my bags. As the fever dragged on, I once again questioned why I had ever left.

Day 6

Sean said the waves looked "fun". I had picked him up the night before in Guadalajara. We rose early, got some food at Denny's (Sean told me I would have to be more careful about what foods I ate for a while until my stomach adjusted.) It was mid-afternoon when we reached La Ticla, A river mouth wave that broke over a cobblestone beach. There was an early season south swell hitting. The size was somewhere overhead high and I saw guys on shortboards making two or three turns before their rides ended.

I disagreed with Sean, I thought the waves looked like scary death waves. Coming straight from the mellow and gentle waves of San Diego, the waves looked anything but fun to me. They looked like monsters, waiting to bitch slap me should I annoy them with my pathetic attempt to slide down their faces. It turned out, we were both right. I watched Sean paddle out, effortlessly duck dive a set and place himself at the peak without ever breathing hard. I grabbed my longboard and managed to get swept four hundred yards down the beach before I ever made it past the white water. After a grueling, thirty-minute paddle battle, I finally made it to sit on my board near Sean. He could see I was already frustrated, and he felt badly for encouraging me to come out in conditions in which I wasn't comfortable. Hooting me into the next medium-sized set wave, he attempted to cheer me up, but failed miserably. I didn't want anything to do with that wave, but he yelled for me to go, thereby letting me have a wave that rightfully belonged to him. I hated it when dudes did that to me! I went, I wiped out. I thought I might die. I surfaced and opened my mouth in a meager attempt to survive, but another wave stacked up. Down I went, back into the black ink. With another two set waves, the current pulled me hundreds of yards down the beach. I was exhausted already, and knew the waves were above my skill level. But my ego wouldn't admit defeat. Sheer determination fueled another ten-minute paddle battle before I made it back out. In the meantime, I saw Sean make three hacks and perfectly kick out of a head- high wave. I was thoroughly pissed at myself. There was no reason he should get good waves while I couldn't. My anger fueled me long enough to get me pummeled two more times before pure exhaustion made me quit.

I climbed the cobblestone beach and sat on a rock to catch my breath. Being a good friend, Sean rode in his next wave. I was crying when he reached me. He found it comical that a bad session could make me cry. It wasn't a bad session that made me cry. I was a bad surfer. I sucked at surfing. I sucked at life. I was a bad human. *What a stupid, ignorant little bitch, Natasha. I was the most arrogant person ever for thinking I could surf in Mexico, and I was a complete fool for coming at all!* Shut up, stupid Voice!

That night food immediately became an issue. The town of La Ticla was really just a few storefronts, a few beachfront restaurants, and a few thatched-roof cabañas for rent for the cost of a decent meal at the Whole Foods buffet back home. For dinner, we walked a block or two into "town". Sean wanted to check on work emails so we found an internet cafe, which I had no idea still existed. The only person to be found inside was a 7-year-old child who was left in charge of the joint. Sean spoke Spanish, thank God. I was shocked that the child was the one in charge, and even seemed to be able to handle the math to make change for Sean. The scene was repeated when a ten-year-old boy was our waiter at a plastic table set up on the shoulder of a dusty street where his mother cooked tacos at a nearby cart. Again, Sean's Spanish saved the day. But it was stressful either way, because the menu consisted of tortillas (carbs, something I didn't eat), cheese (dairy, another "bad" food), and unknown meat (which made me squeamish).

Sean ordered three tacos and a beer. I wanted three tacos and a beer too, but the unwritten food rules state that boys should eat more than girls, and beer had gluten, and gluten is bad. Fumbling through the Spanish, I ordered two tacos and a bottle of water. The tacos were, of course, phenomenal. I savored each bite because the food rules say you should eat more slowly if you are really hungry. I was still hungry after I washed down the second taco with a sip of water. Of course, I was. I was always hungry. But I had eaten my meal and the food rules now dictated that I should wait at least three hours before eating again. Sean commented on how good the tacos were, waving the kid back over.

"Tres mas tacos de carne y una mas corona para me, y para ella...," he questioned me with his face.

WHAT? I was dumbfounded. I understood his words, but their meaning bewildered me. He had just ordered three more tacos and another beer. He ordered seconds...at a restaurant!

And he expected me to do the same!

I fumbled for words, unsure how to respond. Of course, I wanted more food, but that broke the rules. But we had just undergone the same workout. Actually, my session was more strenuous than his...

"Uno mas taco, por favor." I could justify one more.

I sat in silence, savoring every last bit of greasy steak in my taco, being sure to throw away the tortilla (refined carbs are against the food rules), pondering an insane culture in which people ordered seconds at a restaurant. Mind blown!

What happened next befuddled me even further.

Sean once again waved the kid over. I assumed he would ask for the check. Instead, I heard him say, "Uno mas taco de pollo y una Coca." Turning to me, he asked, "You want anything else? How about a beer after all that surfing? You deserve it!"

My jaw dropped. My mind tried to process what had just happened. Not only has Jason ordered a seventh taco, but he ordered a Coke as well. SODA?!?! With HIGH FRUCTOSE CORN SYRUP! And now he was offering me a beer.

I guess he interpreted my confused look as the need for a beer. He told the child to bring us another Corona, too.

I searched for words. Beer. I can't drink beer. Beer has gluten and carbs! My food rules conflicted with my never-say-what-you-really-want-because-someone-might-be-hurt rules. Sean was buying me a beer, and it would be rude to turn down a gift. The deed was done, the beer was ordered. I was going to have to drink that beer!

Ah, I know. I will share it with him. Then I'm only sinning a little. And then I won't eat anymore tonight, and I will surf on an empty stomach in the morning, when the only fuel I have is stored fat. Ok, cool, I can enjoy the beer now without gaining weight.

But then Sean suggested we grab some beers for the cabaña and enjoy the stars and the waves with a six pack. Something didn't add up. Sean was a man in his forties, very fit, not fat at all. How could Sean eat seven tacos and drink soda and beer and look like that? Maybe Sean was on to something.

We went to the corner store, and I searched for the beer cooler while Sean looked for something we could eat in the morning. We met at the counter, me with a variety pack of Mexican beer and Sean with...gulp...a roll of cookies...for breakfast...dun dun DUN!

Cookies for breakfast, Gluten and GMO sugar and artificial ingredients and no protein, for breakfast! I quickly scanned the store and found two bananas and an apple, adding them to the pile on the counter. Still no protein and way too much sugar, but at least better than cookies!

The following morning, I woke before Sean. I was starving. I scarfed down an apple and a banana and went outside, starting to wax the board I wanted to ride. The door cracked open.

"Whoa...do that inside, chica. You're gonna wake up the other surfers with that sound!"

I felt stupid...and hungry.

We surfed that morning, then drove to our next destination. Pasquales. This stop is known by surfers for its big, heavy, barreling waves. We arrived in the evening, just before sunset. The surface was glassy and the waves were living up to their reputation. I saw a female in the lineup, and anxiety gripped me. I had no excuse to stay on the beach if other girls were out on the water.

Sean examined the waves. He concluded that they looked kinda fun, but he was already exhausted from the drive and from surfing that morning. He didn't want to push it, risking injury or illness. The idea that the waves would be good and we had time to surf, but our energy level would prevent us from surfing, shocked me almost as much as eating seven tacos at once. Listening to your body when it is tired? But Sean was a really good surfer. How had he achieved that level without forcing himself to surf every spare moment, no matter how he felt?

In the morning, the waves were no good. Sean conceded that he slightly regretted not surfing the night before. *See! I knew it!* We loaded the car and headed south for Rio Nexpa. After another day of getting beat down while Sean got barreled, and feeling too guilty to eat enough while Sean ate like a king, we finally arrived at a wave that looked like heaven to me: Saladita.

Day 9

Sean didn't bother paddling out. He handed me my longboard and told me to go enjoy a victory lap. The waves were knee to waist high and broke to the surfers left for hundreds of yards. As I paddled out I watched surfers run to the nose of their big boards and stand there with backs arched and hands behind the back. It was like the famous wave in California, Malibu, only in reverse. The lineup was equally similar to Malibu, crowded and unfriendly. I was confident in waves this size. I paddled to the peak and quickly found a wave to call my own. But before I knew it two other people thought they should share the wave with me. I shouted at them to let them know I was behind them and they should make their exit ASAP. The surfer directly in front of me turned around and looked at me as if I was a freak. She hollered back at me,

"You can't call someone off a wave unless you can catch up to them!" Just then the white water that she had caused from her drop-in caught up to me and I was knocked from my board. A few other women gave me the stink eye when I caught my next few waves. Eventually, I paddled in to find Sean sipping a cold beer in the shade.

"Well," he asked, "How was it?"

"What am I doing here? Any wave I'm good enough to surf is overrun by bitchy white girls who think they own the place!" I didn't feel unique or brave for doing what I was doing. I felt like a cliche.

"You'll find your wave, and you'll rise to the occasion, just give yourself some time."

I didn't believe him. We reloaded the boards and set off ten miles down the road to my final destination, Troncones.

Sean helped me unload all my stuff into my new home. It was twice the size of my San Diego apartment, had an ocean view, a deck for doing yoga, and a gorgeous jacuzzi tub. Perhaps the Mexican life would be a lot better than I had anticipated.

Next order of business: check out the waves. On our way down to the beach, we passed a beautiful pool with a swim-up bar. Several people lounged there. Every one of them was over sixty and speaking English. A super nice, heavyset woman introduced herself, offering to share a package of doughnuts with me. Bright white bodies glistening with sunscreen filled the lounge chairs around the pool.

I had imagined that I'd be staying at a surfer's hotel. I had envisioned a fresh truckload of guys in board shorts and flat-billed hats coming in with each new swell. I would never have admitted to it, but I also envisioned a lot of under the radar flings with said surfer dudes after epic sessions in the water. Knowing I would never see them again, I could have a new man every week if I wanted.

"Where do you think all the other surfers are?" I asked Sean.

"Maybe in the water?" he replied hopefully.

We rounded the pool to look out over the ocean. It was flat, like a lake.

"Maybe it's between sets?" He was still trying to be optimistic.

One guy sat, motionless, atop a longboard next to the point where the waves should have been. Other than him, the water was empty. We waited and watched. Eventually, a tiny ripple popped up. The man on the longboard paddled as hard as he could for fifteen yards before finally standing up. The wave abruptly mushed out and the ride ended as soon as it started.

"Maybe the swell just isn't hitting here at the right angle?" Sean suggested. He could see clearly that I was crestfallen.

We made our way back to my apartment, passing the doughnut-eating American retirees. I plopped down on the bed, and Sean sat beside me. I had just rearranged my entire life to come stay at the equivalent of Winter Haven Florida, where my retired grandparents owned a trailer home to escape the northern winters.

Sean finally broke the silence.

"You can't stay here."

"But I committed to it. They are planning on me." I felt trapped. Just the thought of bailing out on my commitment made me feel sick with guilt, and hungry.

"You are on a surf trip. You want to surf three times a day. You don't owe anyone anything. You can still say no."

The concept blew my mind. I could say no. I could change my mind. I could do whatever I wanted. I didn't have to stay and suffer. I could end it. I wasn't trapped. I sat in silence.

"You can't stay here," he repeated.

He was right. I was going to be miserable. I was going to resent the people to whom I was supposed to be showing hospitality. If I didn't take care of myself first, I would end up causing more harm than good. And the whole point of the trip was to take care of myself.

It felt shallow and scary. It felt shallow because I wanted waves and romance, but these people had offered me a job. My values told me hard work was good but sex and recreation were bad. It felt scary because I didn't have much money. I had just left my whole life behind only to have no plan at all. It felt like I was free falling.

Still overwhelmed with guilt, the following morning I talked to the manager. I informed him I would not be staying. As soon as the conversation was over, I lit up with energy at the release of the emotional weight. After a boat trip to nearby secret reef break, I dropped off Sean at the airport that afternoon. I was on my own, with absolutely no plan, no income, no companion, and unable to speak the language. I cried when he left, scared to be alone. But I quickly stanched the tears. I reminded myself that this was an adventure, all experiences were welcome.

Not knowing what else to do I returned to the longboard wave, hoping I had just been there on a crowded day. There, I immediately encountered a group of local surfer boys who were more than happy to help me locate accommodations. More than happy, once they realized I was a single female traveling alone. They also invited me to have a beer and eat a fish they had just caught. Just like that, my entire attitude shifted.

Chapter 21: Saladita

Days 11-25

I sat in an empty restaurant waiting for someone called "El Jefe". It was dark under the thatched palm roof. The floor was made of sand. The wife and daughter of El Jefe waited with me. They had just informed me that my cabaña would be $30 per night. But I knew every penny I spent was limiting the time I could spend traveling. It was the cheapest I had found, but still out of my budget. I asked if maybe there was some work I could do to help pay for my room. Apparently "The Boss" was going to have to discuss that one with me. I tried my best to make small talk but I struggled, writing down a lot of words to look up later. Soon an old man wearing cowboy boots, a rancher's hat, with a huge grey handlebar mustache showed up. He sat across the table from me and looked at me like I was lost. Then he asked me a single question. He spoke slowly. His words carried importance.
"Te Gusta Donald Trump?"
"No," I burst out laughing. "No es mi presidente! Por eso estoy aquí."
It satisfied him. Then the wife arraigned for me to help in the restaurant for four hours each Sunday afternoon. In exchange, I would be given a $10 reduction in rent per night. I was stoked and also terrified. I had no idea how I was going to work in a restaurant with my limited Spanish. I paid for two weeks upfront, informing the landlord that I intended to stay for a minimum of one month. At least, that's what I thought I told him, in Spanish. I was still concerned about how I would afford $20 per night, plus food, since I hadn't planned to spend any money during the duration of my previous work

trade arrangement. But I had other things on my mind at that point. Boys and surfing!

After two days, I found an open-air palapa with a concrete floor perfect for doing yoga. I tracked down the owner and, a bottle of whisky in hand, I used my best formal Spanish to request permission to hold yoga classes in his palapa. I spread the word to the surfers that I would be teaching classes daily at noon. For the next two weeks, I constantly had six to eight yoga students, who donated enough to pay for my food, rent, and gasoline for the day. After another week, a friend from Facebook contacted me. She was a yoga instructor and massage therapist at a high-end yoga retreat in a nearby resort town. She was about to go on vacation and wanted to know if I might sub for her for a couple of weeks, while she was away. On Sundays, I waited tables and learned how to make authentic guacamole. I learned the words for broom, onion, octopus, and a lot more, very quickly. The cook took a liking to me and kept me constantly fed.

I had been scared to move out of the house with Kurt because I might run out of money. I had been scared to leave my yoga studio because I might run out of money. I had been scared to leave my original work-trade agreement at the retirement resort because I might run out of money. Taking each step away from what didn't serve me required me to completely give up control. It took blind faith in the idea that acting in my best interests could only lead to something better. And now, here I was, one week in a new country and already had three jobs that paid more than the one I'd left, back in California.

The surfing did turn out to be fun after I figured out which sections were easiest to catch waves, learned the pecking order, and made a couple of allies with some of the expat local women. I was even invited to a birthday party where I spent the night getting drunk and thinking my Spanish was flawless. I was beginning to feel like I fit in.

Then there was the issue of attention from men. Although I had yet to admit it, I knew it was one of the main reasons I had come on this trip--to have casual sex with men I would never see again. I wanted to forget Kurt was ever in my life. I wanted to have a life far more exciting, far bigger, than he could have ever given me. And for the first time ever, to be in full control of my sexuality without guilt. Mexican men are incredible sweet talkers and pursue women aggressively. Even better for me, they really love the female body, in any size, shape, or form. The men found me something of a novelty, given that I am tall and was becoming quite plump. Throw in a big helping of machismo, and I was hooked. The first guy was a local surf instructor. He took me surfing under the full moon. I watched in awe as bioluminescence sprayed off our surfboards. After the session we stood in the midnight heat, rinsing off the salt water with a bucket. We sprinted, naked and giggling, across the beach back to my cabaña.

Boundaries became an issue for me. I just wanted attention and sex, but marrying an American girl offered life-changing potential to a local. As soon as I slept with the surf instructor, it was as if he thought we were spouses and soul mates. He wanted every moment of my time. I have always enjoyed a rhythm to my day. It frazzles me to give away too much personal time. I found it very difficult to shoo him away when I wanted my space. It seemed un-nice. And I cared way too much about hurting someone's feelings to be having that kind of casual sex. I couldn't keep him away from me. I didn't feel like fucking all the time and I didn't want to have to coddle his feelings. That left only one other option, leave. I was scared. But it didn't take long before I knew I had to move on. I was on an adventure. Drama has always been my drug, and life was getting too easy. I grew bored of perfect little longboard waves, craving something more exciting. I was spending most of each day at the yoga retreat, working. I knew I hadn't come to Mexico to work. I had come to surf. I arrived home from work one night to the landlady, who explained to me that she had rented my place to someone else who was willing to pay more. I would either need to outbid him or move along.

I was terrified to drive alone through Mexico, terrified to be without a paycheck, terrified to surf more challenging waves. But I knew my heart wanted to keep moving, and I knew enough to trust my desires. They hadn't steered me wrong yet.

Plan A was to stay at the retirement resort. I revised that plan when I saw how unhappy it would make me, even though abandoning its certainty was scary. Plan B, staying at the mellow longboard spot and earning some money by teaching yoga, was also falling through. Plan C was no plan at all, perhaps just to continue driving, seeing what might turn up. But the idea of driving alone in Mexico, without a destination, seemed incredibly irresponsible.

On my last night staying in the little surf village, I put my headphones on and went for a walk under the stars. In the morning, I would need to figure out my next move. I walked near the shoreline, where the waves met the beach, and let cool water splash on my legs, contrasting the warmth of the night. Nearly full, the moon was perfectly clear, with a million trillion stars lighting up the sky.

I had done it. I had escaped from hell. But, even as I bathed in the moonlight, in the most heavenly setting imaginable, my heart ached for the loss of my marriage. I began to cry as the pain of losing my husband bubbled up once again. It had been five and a half months since I filed for divorce. In just a couple of weeks, it would be final. Knowing I would be on the road in some mysterious land lacking proper internet connections meant my decision was final. I was letting him go, for good. And look at what I had created for myself without him--the adventure of a lifetime. Kesha filled my headphones as I walked the moonlit coast, her every word seeming to issue from my heart into Kurt's.

Well, you almost had me fooled,
told me that I was nothing without you.
But after everything you've done,
I can thank you for how strong I have become.
Cuz you brought the flames and you put me through hell.
I had to learn how to fight for myself,
and we both know all the truth I could tell.
I'll just say this is I wish you farewell

Water caressed on my legs. Moonlight touched my sunburnt skin. Whitewater formed perfect, surfable lines.

I hope your soul is changing,
I hope you find your peace,
falling on your knees praying.
Someday maybe you will see the light.

Tears streamed down my cheeks, and I began to run.

I'm proud of who I am.
No more monsters, I can breathe again.
And you said that I was done.
Well, you were wrong and now the best is yet to come.
Cuz I can make it on my own.

I ran harder, faster, and started screaming the lyrics. The farther I ran, the faster my strides. My heart beat into the red zone, but I didn't care. Sprinting and screaming, racing alone down the empty beach, my chest threatened to explode. My toe caught and I pitched forward, belly-flopping onto the soft, wet sand. I sat, heaving and sobbing, as a wave surged in and soaked me up to my chest. Still, Kesha's words rang out as if straight from my own heart.

*I found a strength I've never known
When I'm finished they won't even know your name.*

Sopping wet, I picked myself up and found a palm tree a few feet from the breaking waves. Leaning against the palm, I opened a new note in my phone and began to write:

Dear Kurt,

I hope one day we will have the kind of relationship where I can give you this letter. But if that never happens, I will be okay. I loved you so hard, and I lost so hard. I am already okay, I am more than okay. I am amazing. I wanted to thank you. I didn't know life could get this good. Today I surfed 5 hours in the most beautiful palm tree paradise you can imagine. You'd love it here. Nose rides for days. My only problem in life today is that there is so much more life to experience. I am happy, no really, I am. And I owe this to you.

Thank you for taking me surfing when I was first learning, for taking me to your shaper and helping me get a custom board. Thank you for teaching me how to buy a proper fitting wetsuit and how to wax a board and how to install fins and how to tie the board to the roof of my car. Thank you for showing me the surf spots around our home and quizzing me on their names. Thanks for introducing me to surf culture and the surfing forefathers and surf history and surfboard evolution. Thanks for making me read articles in Surfer's Journal that you knew were important. Thanks for making me watch surf movies to help with my style. Thanks for taking me to Mexico for my first time and getting me to the proper waves so I could learn to go directional. Thanks for showing me how to travel in Mexico, how to get around, and teaching me not to be afraid. Thanks for never, ever criticizing. Thanks for being patient with me when I cried on clean-up set waves. Thanks for not over-coaching me, but giving me room to learn at my own pace.

Thanks for not encouraging me even when I was surfing good, it made me work harder.

And you know what else? Thanks for not complimenting my body when I craved your attention, thanks for not touching my leg under the table when we sat next to each other, thanks for never holding my hand, thanks for sitting on the opposite couch as me every night and zoning out to the TV. Thanks for never saying I looked beautiful when I put on a dress. Thanks for never grabbing my ass or stealing a kiss when I walked by.

Thank you for saying I was fat. Thank you for crushing my self-esteem. No really, there is no sarcasm or bitterness here, I mean it, thank you.

You gave me the gift of misery. You withheld outside validation. I craved your compliments and your touch. Without them, my ego became needier and needier to the point where I could not take it anymore. Without you to medicate my poor self-esteem I was forced to feel all the pain, to walk through the suffering, to wallow in the discomfort. You made my darkest self come out.

And I found that victory was waiting for me on the other side. One million of your compliments and loving touches would have never been enough. I looked to your love to fill me, and when I didn't receive it, I was forced to look within. That is the greatest gift anyone could have ever given me.

I tried to fix you. Just like I tried to fix Josh, just like my mom tried to fix me. I made subtle suggestions, I did things for you that you could have done for yourself, I made sure you knew I was smarter than you. I assumed that if you would just do everything the way I told you to do it that all would be well in the world.

And then you threw it all in my face with a big FUCK YOU the day you went and got high for the first time in almost seven years. You forced me to drag my codependent, manipulative, better-than-you self to al-anon where they held up a mirror to showed me my disease was as active as yours. I learned to give up control over you, and everyone else. I learned that people don't need me. I learned that the only one who needs fixing is myself. You, my dear qualifier, you taught me that.

And oh My Love, you taught me to fight. Dear Water Blue Eyed Lover, it was you who made me strong! I was weak and unsure of myself. You sent me to therapy where I learned to set boundaries. Your temper broke me free of the spell of co-dependence. The moment that glazed look came over my soul mate's face and a monster spoke through my best friend's mouth, I learned to detach with love. You, my Very Best Friend in the whole wide world, taught me how to love unconditionally. Because of you, I wanted to die. You drove me to the darkest moments of my life and because of YOU, my Dream Man, my Partner, I found out what I was made of. I found out I was made of the stuff of stars. I am force, I am the very breath of God. You, my Big Strong Man, you drove me into my shit, into the depths where I found bedrock and there, on rock-solid truth, I set my anchors firm at last. Because of you, My Heart's Truest Love, I am unshakable. Nothing can separate me from who I know I am.

I am un-fuckable-with.

I have the strength of the universe. I can do anything. And I will.

I will do everything.

You, Kurt, you set me on fire. Thank you, thank you, thank you.
With unconditional gratitude,
Your Wife

And I meant it. Every word of it.

The Kesha song was on repeat for about the fourteenth time.

Well you almost had me fooled
I had to learn how to fight for myself
I hope you find your peace
I'm proud of who I am
I found a strength I've never known
The best is yet to come!

The next morning, I packed my truck once more and made my way to Mex-200. I turned right, toward the south, toward the unknown.

Chapter 22: Acapulco

Day 26

With absolutely no plan except to look for surf, I set off to the Land of Deeper. The farther south I traveled, the more rural and wild the land became. Just before I departed the mellow longboard spot, a friend of mine gave me a puppy she had rescued from a starving, sickly mother who was trying to survive while nursing nine puppies in the jungle.

"Here, you are going to need a little protection on your trip," she said, handing me the most docile, three-month-old puppy I'd ever seen. I plopped the little thing in the passenger seat, where she promptly fell asleep. *Some protection.* The poor little girl could hardly lift her head. I named her Mika, and I couldn't stop smiling each time I looked over at her droopy face.

A couple of hours passed as I cruised south, listening to podcasts, slamming on my brakes each time topes (Mexican speed bumps) appeared out of nowhere. I flipped through my guidebook, which laid out all the surfing spots in Mainland Mexico. The spots were depicted from north to south, with brief descriptions of how to find the waves and what to expect in each area. The guidebook listed a break coming up, but warned that it was near a drug trafficking town where you were likely to get ripped off if you left your vehicle unattended. I could see the turnoff for the surfing spot approaching, about a hundred yards ahead. I slowed, but decided it wasn't worth checking out. But as I looked up I saw that just beyond the turnoff, a tree lay across both lanes of Mex-200. A large, jacked-up, black truck was parked next to the tree.

OH CRAP OH CRAP OH CRAP

I knew instantly what was up. No one has nice, jacked-up trucks in the middle of rural Mexico-- unless they are cartel. And no one hangs out next to freshly cut trees in the middle of the road unless they are trying to clear them, which these people were not, or they don't want you to pass. There was no other way around the tree, on the only road for hundreds of miles. This was a roadblock.

I made a quick decision and a hard, right-hand turn. *Maybe I'll go surfing after all!* After a mile or so, the dirt road dead-ended at a right-hand point break. No surfers were out, just as the guide book predicted. I tied my puppy to the truck, grabbed a surfboard and paddled out, hoping I could wait out the road blockers.

The waves were messy, it appeared the swell was too small and the direction wasn't well lined up for the spot. I got a couple of short rides that quickly faded out to nothing. I kept thinking I heard my dog barking, back on the beach. I was completely paranoid and shaking. The surf session was worthless. I took a wave in and found my car untouched, my dog napping quietly in the shade, water bowl untouched. I stood there, staring at her, staring at my truck, staring back out toward the road. I considered my options. I could take my chances and hope the road was cleared, or I could turn around and go back to the place I had just left. But that would mean the end of my adventure, and I would have to go back to working to be able to afford the more expensive rent and food in that area. No, I was on a surf trip, a grand adventure. Kesha words still filled my head, "I can make it on my own. I found a strength I've never known." Onward and deeper!

I got in the car and put the windows down to let out the 120-degree heat before loading up my puppy, Mika, and the boards. I made a U-turn and headed back up the dirt road toward the highway. *God, please let them be gone when I get back!* Mika was sleeping again. *Geeze, does she know how to do anything else?* I turned the music off as I slowly navigated the washed-out road. Up ahead, I could see the paved road. It was decision time. To the left, back to safety, a job, crappy waves, the familiar, control? Or to the right, toward danger, risk, the unknown, freedom?

I turned right.

As soon as I turned, I regretted it. The tree was still there. The truck was still there. The doors to the truck were flung open, and two men wearing bandanas over their faces jumped out, each man brandishing an assault rifle.
OH CRAP OH CRAP OH CRAP!
I activated the automatic window, but it crept upward at the speed of a lazy snail. The men were running, making a beeline for my car. The window was too slow, too slow, too slow! Mika lifted her head. Sensing my fear, she stood to her feet in the passenger seat for the first time.

The men reached my car and the upward progress of my window was halted by the cold barrel of an AR-15, held at eye level.
"Baja la ventana!" They screamed at me. I knew they wanted me to open the window but I pretended not to understand.

"I don't speak Spanish." I replied, "No Espanol!" I lifted my hands and shook my head. I lied; it had been over three weeks and I had learned survival Spanish by that time.

The first guy tried the door handle and then pounded on the door when he found it was locked. There was no pretending I didn't understand that gesture. I opted for the lesser of two evils and rolled down the window. The man stuck his head in the window and looked at the surf equipment and dirty clothing strewn about the back. He looked back to me, then reached for my sunglasses, which were perched on my head.

"No!" Some unknown courage came over me as I ducked away. "Get your hands off of me! Deja me sola" I yelled with some kind of confidence that wasn't my own. I had learned the phrase from one of the ex-pat girls I met after yoga last week. She said it was useful for the men. He seemed shocked and he did as he was told, backing away. The second man stuck his head in my window, performed a similar inventory, and then pointed at my iPhone, laid between the seats.

"No!" I said again, this time sounding more annoyed than fierce.

"Si!" the man replied and started to reach over me.

Just as the man's hand was part way into the window, my sleepy little puppy let out the most pathetic bark I've ever heard and jumped into my lap, knocking down the hand reaching over me. It was enough. The man pulled his hand back. He looked annoyed.

"¿A donde vas? ¿Estas sola?"

He was asking me where I was going and if I was alone.

"Surfing," I replied, ignoring the question as to whether I was alone.

He eyed me, lowered his gun, and started laughing. I really don't know why.

"Hay un impuesto, quinientos pesos." He said there was a tax of about twenty-five US dollars.

I returned his laugh, though I had no idea why we were laughing. I made a show of searching all over the truck for some cash. I finally handed him the equivalent of $12. I made sure to use my worst gringa accent as I told him in Spanish that I didn't have any more money. He asked if I had any water. I said yes and handed him a large bottle. He asked if I needed directions or a cabaña rental for the night. I said no. He told me to have a nice day. Both men slung their guns on their backs, walked slowly back to the tree, moved it from the road, and proceeded to wave me through. I smiled and waved and trembled as I continued on my merry little way.

I put Kesha back on the radio. "I can make it on my own..." And slowly the shaking stopped.

Day 27-41

As the sunset on my first day of solo driving, I located a tiny town in which my book indicated there were surfing waves. I found a small hotel--really, just a large house with extra rooms. I negotiated a price of $20 for the night, parked the truck behind the gate, and set out on foot in search of food and waves. I found a beach, but the ocean was flat. A man emerged from a beachfront home to inquire what the strange, big white girl was doing there. He spoke a little English and was happy to practice with me. I told him I wanted to go surfing. He laughed. He said the surfing season wasn't for three more months. I asked him if there was any place to eat. He said there were no restaurants in town, but there was a store where I could buy food.

Panic rose at the thought of having to go to bed without a hot dinner. Control...I had none. I pushed down the fear and searched for the store. When I found the store, my panic only increased. It was your typical Mexican corner store, filled with cookies and soda but not much else. I bought a package of crackers, a Diet Coke, and some brownies that appeared to be homemade. No workout for the day, chocolate for dinner, I felt my butt getting bigger before I even walked out the door. Luckily, I found some children playing soccer in the street. They let me join them for long enough to work up a sweat, whereby I regained a bit of control. I felt at least a bit more justified in polishing off the last of my processed food.

The next surf spot in my book was a suburb, just outside Acapulco. I'd probably make it there by lunchtime. Entering the city limits, I noticed my car driving a little funny. It wasn't shifting very easily into drive from the park, and it was struggling to climb the hills. The speedometer didn't budge when I stepped on the gas, but the RPM's jumped instead. OH CRAP.

I pulled over once again to do the only two things I knew how to do: check the fluids and call my Dad.

"It sounds like the transmission, hon. You better get to a mechanic." My Dad didn't have any better news for me.

Once again, The Voice began to scold me. *I was an idiot for ever leaving California. I was going to run out of money. Why hadn't I stayed in Troncones, where I had a good job and okay waves?*

"No WAY. I'm in this! There is nothing I can't handle." I spoke out loud, and to my surprise, it worked. The Voice shut up, supplanted by a second, more helpful voice.

"You are so badass! You totally got this! Who cares what happens? It's all part of the adventure. BOOM POW YEAH!" This new voice sounded like a fat African American woman. I liked her voice a lot.

Strategically, I chose a mechanic on the same street as the surfing beach. After a challenging bit of communication, I learned that my transmission would need to be rebuilt, and that the repairs would take five days. The mechanic had a sort of mother-in-law house and said he would rent it to me while I waited for the car to be fixed.

My room was $5 per night. There was no AC and only one window. The room was built of concrete. It resembled a prison cell. The cell housed two sets of bunk beds and two queen beds, all equipped with bare, brown-and-green striped mattresses. I knew exactly where the dingy, piss-stained mattresses had come from, because I'd previously seen Mexican men cruising the allies in San Diego neighborhoods, reclaiming them from spots alongside dumpsters. I saw trucks full of these beds, objects that homeless people and feral dogs used to call home. I saw them stacked in the back of trucks, cruising down Interstate 5, heading toward the Tijuana border. And now, I was paying to sleep on one of them, rusty springs jabbing my back all night long. Electricity was supplied to my prison cell via an extension cable running from the landlord's house into mine. I could plug in a light, a fan, and my phone charger. The toilet had no seat, but it flushed. The shower had no hot water, but it had water. With no control over my car, my living situation, or my length of stay, somehow I was totally content.

I had been staying in the suburb, Playa Bonfil, waiting on my car's repairs for three days. I had spent two terrifying surf sessions in overhead waves that broke with the force of freeway collisions. This was a beach break. Instead of the wave breaking predictably over a reef they broke on shifting sandbars. The best beach break surfers have a way of reading the rips and knowing where the next set will show up. I was far from the best. These waves were massive slabs. One moment they were nothing but a bump on the surface of the ocean and the next they were turning themselves inside out, towering way above your head, throwing the lip way out in front of them, leaving a hollow cavern inside. I was just learning to shortboard, and was taking frequent heavy wipeouts. The paddle back to the line-up was always brutal. Having to duck dive under sets, often having my board ripped from my hands, then looking up to see another wave about to dump right over me, drilling me underwater before I had a chance for a proper breath. I would be exhausted and terrified each and every time I made it out the back. I hadn't seen another girl in the line-up yet, and I wouldn't see another girl for ten more days. I never saw another white person, and I never heard a word of English spoken on the water. My sun-and-salt-bleached-blond hair and female body parts were an instant sensation. Which, of course, I loved.

The heavy beach break and the charming locals quickly grew on me. I'm not sure what I liked more, catching waves or watching guys try to catch me after surfing. The local surfers at Playa Bonfil called themselves the Bonfil Boys and Team Radical. They could shred, for sure, some of the best surfing I've seen anywhere in the world. The waves lent themselves to both barrel riding and aerial maneuvers. As I walked the beach to paddle out, someone would hoot at me from a palapa. As I paddled for a wave, someone would hoot at me, "Da'le Güara! Da'le!" (Go white girl, go!). Post-surf sessions were the best. The boys would gather at a beachside restaurant with a perfect view of the waves to have breakfast, beers and share stories. Although my Spanish sucked and I struggled to say anything meaningful, I was always hooted at to join them. Post-surf beers would turn into photoshoots, where each and every boy wanted a picture with me, wanted to put his arm around my hips (which met the height of his ribs), or wanted to tag me in a Facebook photo. I was invited to a party in town. I was invited to go wake surfing. I was invited to the movies. I was invited out for micheladas. If I walked through town, each time I crossed an intersection someone down the road would yell, "Natashaaaa". I was popular.

One evening, I sat in my jail cell of an apartment, the door cracked so my puppy, Mika, could go in and out. The dog was teething and had a bad habit of chewing everything. I was a new dog owner and had a bad habit of never watching her. While I played a language game on my phone, Mika found the extension cable that ran power to my unit. It must have tasted good, because I heard a blood-curdling yelp from outside the door--and the lights went out. I ran outside to pull the poor little thing off of the cord, the current so strong that she couldn't remove herself. It zapped me pretty good through her limp body. I screamed, scooped up my baby, and started crying.

A female scream in a run-down Mexican neighborhood is a call to action. The twenty-two-year-old boy who lived next door leaped over my locked gate in about 7.3 seconds. Within thirty seconds, several more young men had found their way into my gated and locked yard. I tried to explain, through sign language and awful Spanish, what had happened. One of the guys figured out that I was without power, and he sprang to address the problem. Without unplugging the cable, he proceeded to fix the exposed wire, using a rock to shave back the insulation. With some plastic ripped from his baggy of weed, he insulated his hand while he spliced the wires back together. Borrowing a piece of used electrical tape from another spot on the cable, he sealed up the whole job. Good as new. I had light, and new friends.

The guys wanted to show me around the city. I didn't know them, and these fence jumpers didn't exactly seem like stand up guys. I could hardly communicate with them. The Voice told me what a good girl *should* do. But the good girl also should never have left San Diego, should never have gotten a divorce, and shouldn't eat bad food. She most definitely shouldn't go out with young, strange men in the middle of the night in one of the world's most dangerous cities. Screw it! Acapulco turns out to be a wonderful place to party.

The boys always say they are 25. But I asked around, and I'm pretty sure the guy who had taken the most liking to me was closer to 21. He didn't speak a word of English and I had only about 100 words of Spanish. He was employed by the mechanic who was rebuilding my transmission. He kept coming around after that night. For a few days, I resisted him. I liked his company but I wasn't very attracted to him. Finally, I wrote in my journal, *I think I'm going to let him fuck me soon. Why not? I'm sure his youthful energy will be fun!*

One night the mechanic, the lover boy, and I all went out downtown. We picked up the mechanic's mistress and spent the night dancing, eating tacos, and swimming in the ocean at 4:00 am. I somehow lost all my clothes on the beach and had to wear a lover boy's tank top like a dress, sneaking back into my hotel at dawn. That morning I told my journal, *I think I just had the best night of my life.*

Guilt-free sex felt like getting out of prison. But, as with the surf instructor, I had trouble shutting the door I had opened. The case with lover boy was even more difficult because I had no Spanish vocabulary for being nice. I knew how to say, "Leave me alone." But it was too difficult to say, "I really like you and I think you are a wonderful person, it's just that I value my alone time and I really don't have an appetite for sex at this moment, so please don't take this personally, I'd appreciate some space and I'll call you as soon as I get horny again." Instead, I just slept with him a few more times. He was young and did his business rather quickly. I could return to my own schedule after a few minutes, feeling just a bit icky inside. I was reminded of what my friend Stephanie (a professional at one night stands) had once told me:

"Nat, sometimes you gotta just find your inner bitch. A polite no might as well be a yes!"

Although that's pretty messed up, she was right. But I had a long way to go before I found my blunt-voiced inner bitch.

In Acapulco, I realized that practically no one saw my body like I did. All of the attention made me feel like a supermodel. I loosened my food rules. The journey to honoring my hunger had begun in San Diego more than a year earlier, and I now ate consistently when I felt hunger. But eating enough to feel satisfied, without labeling some foods as bad and others as good, was still too advanced for me.

Leaving my food safety zone was nerve-racking. Everything in Mexico was fried in lard, covered in cheese, and wrapped in a tortilla. But I didn't eat grains, saturated fat, or dairy, because everyone "knows" those are bad for you. I needed at least a hundred grams of protein per day, I told myself. A few measly pieces of chicken in my taco weren't going to cut it. I would certainly lose muscle if I didn't get more protein. Maybe a little dairy would be okay--there is protein in dairy, after all. Maybe Mexican dairy had fewer hormones. Maybe the corn in the tortillas wasn't GMO, and it wouldn't be quite so bad if I just ate one or two. Maybe...oh my gosh! I could feel my thighs getting fatter with each forbidden bite.

Most restaurants didn't have the "healthy" foods I cooked for myself back home. Even if they featured the correct ingredients, I lacked the Spanish vocabulary to make special requests. Plus, it seemed rude and culturally insensitive to ask the cook to change her homemade specialty just for me. That would contradict my "always be nice" rule. So I started to loosen up.

I was fatter than I had ever been in my life, and had more attention than ever before. I realized for the first time that sexiness was an internal feeling, rather than a number on the scale. With all the attention reassuring me I wasn't disgusting, I cared much less about what I ate. I started eating foods I had previously considered bad. I also allowed myself to eat until I was full. I didn't see it at the time, but the link between the attention from men and my ability to nourish myself was strong. I felt loved just as I was, so I gave myself permission to be who I am. Attention that I had previously considered shallow and felt guilty for seeking was exactly what I needed to nourish my starving soul. My desires were healthy after all.

I met Raul on the evening of my fourth day in town. I was eating at a streetside cafe when one of the tallest Mexicans I'd ever seen started dodging cars, sprinting across the highway, making a beeline for me. Raul spoke English and I was relieved to have an actual conversation for the first time in several days.

"You were surfing this morning, right?" He must have spotted me in the lineup. I didn't recognize him. I always loved it when that happened.

"Yeah…" I responded hesitantly. What did this six-foot-three, two hundred pound guy want from me?
"I wanted to give you something."

He had with him a copy of Surfer Magazine from last year and two bars of wax, one pink and one green. The magazine had obviously changed hands many times, and I would not be the final owner either. Raul pulled up a chair and asked if he was bothering me. I told him no, and we chatted for a while. I asked him how he found me eating dinner that night.

"Amiga, you are blond, you are white, you are big. Have you seen anyone else like you? Be careful, amiga. A lot of guys will do a lotta things to be around you."

His words were meant to caution me, but instead, they excited me. I wasn't physically attracted to him but he was fun and I enjoyed running around town with him. Raul kept trying to buy me things and take me places. I knew he had money because I knew he sold drugs. But I also knew his gifts came with obligation. Once, I let him hijack an entire day for which I had other plans, albeit plans simply to go for a run and do yoga. Like most of the guys I met, Raul was persistent and very difficult to deny. A polite "no" might as well have been an enthusiastic "yes". By the end of the day, we found ourselves in a pool, sipping beers. His hand crept up my leg. A gentle touch to my inner thigh is my kryptonite.

Raul had already tried to grab me and kiss me many times, and I had always refused him. This time, his touch sent a little jolt of electricity through my lady parts. Though I didn't want to be, I was physically stimulated. I asked him to stop, but he sensed that my will was weakening.

"Let me just do this for you. You don't have to give me anything in return." His finger slipped slightly under the edge of my bikini bottoms.

I argued with him, protesting that it didn't seem fair, because I already knew I wasn't going to do anything in return.

"Don't worry so much," he soothed. "Just the pleasure of your company today and getting to touch you is all I want."

I let my body relax as his fingers brought me satisfaction. But as soon as my moans quieted, his dick was out and homing toward me.

"Whoa!" I stopped him. For one thing, he wasn't using a condom, and for another, I wasn't attracted to him. I didn't want to do that. I consciously reminded myself that I did not have to have sex for fear of not being liked or out of obligation. My boundary-setting muscles were strengthening.

He lost his shit and cursed me out. How unfair of me not to return the favor! I wish I could say that I slapped him and walked away, but I hadn't grown that strong yet. I defended myself and my actions. He didn't see it my way. The argument persisted for 15 minutes. I couldn't stand the fact that he might be mad at me. Clearly, casual sexual behavior would yet require more self- confidence.

After a few weeks in Acapulco, binging at the buffet of male attention, the road beckoned with its promise of new adventures.

I heard whispers of an island accessible only by boat, blessed with great waves. I was told that local families rented cabañas on the beach, and opened their homes to serve food to the handful of backpackers and traveling surfers who found their way there. My guidebook listed the surf break as well, but warned that the road to the boat launch was washed out and only accessible by 4x4. It seemed like an invitation. I packed up and headed deeper south. The further south I traveled, the wilder things became, the more my confidence was tested.

Chapter 23: Island Paradise

Day 42-48

Five hours after leaving Acapulco, I encountered a small sign, pointing down a dirt road off the main highway. The sign bore the name of the town I wanted to find. I pulled over to check my map. This seemed to be it. A little old lady waved at me from a corner store. I waved back. She picked up her woven basket, full of market purchases, and headed for my passenger door. She opened the door and hopped in. *Apparently, waving at old ladies gets you hitchhikers in this town.* My Spanish was still pretty basic, but I was pretty sure she said she lived in the town where the boats were launched to go to the legendary island. She said the road was passable, and she would show me the way. Score!

When I dropped off La Abuela, she insisted I sit for a while in her hammock. She showed me around her homestead, a thatched-roof bamboo hut and a yard full of dogs and chickens. She gave me avocados from her yard as a thank you, and directions to the boat launch. I began to treasure these small interactions I had with the Mexican people. It seemed that in culture without Uber, without Yelp Reviews, without even yellow pages, that relationships became a sort of business necessity. If you wanted to survive in this rugged place you had to build a community. Keeping to yourself, doing your own thing, being an individual wasn't strong, it was foolish.

As I pulled up to the launch, several young men waved me into parking areas, hustling for boat clients. I went with the first one, parking behind the gate. I was informed that my car and belongings would be watched, 24/7, at a price of $2 per day. At least that is what I thought he said. I hoped I wasn't about to get all my stuff ripped off. I asked if there was surfing on the island, but I couldn't comprehend the response. I asked if there were accommodations on the island, and understood none of that answer, either. I thought my Spanish had improved from my two English-free weeks in Acapulco but I was extremely frustrated now. I would later find out that the beautiful dark-skinned islanders spoke an afro-influenced dialect. They were impossible for me to understand. I tried asking another kid, but again found the reply unintelligible.

So, I grabbed all three of my boards, camera gear, dog food, and a backpack. I loaded the tiny ponga with way too much stuff. We made the crossing and I paid the $0.75 toll as I was dumped on the shore with a pile of bags, a yapping puppy, and no clue what to do next--or if I was even in the right place. I loaded myself up like a sherpa and headed across the soft sand, carrying a hundred pounds of gear and the dog (the sand was too hot for her paws), pushing through sweltering heat.

I crested a dune, sweat dripping into my wide eyes. BOOM! There, on the other side of the beach, a massive, perfectly formed, hollow wave raced before me. The winds were blowing straight offshore, the good direction. Only two surfers inhabited the water. An uncrowded hollow wave almost doesn't exist anymore. My heart raced. I continued my trek across the beach, arms so full I was unable to swat at the mosquitos who undoubtedly smelled fresh gringa meat and swarmed around my legs. Finding a clump of cabañas, I dumped my stuff in front of the first one. The proprietor came out to negotiate a price with me. I had no idea what she was saying. It might as well have been Arabic. I was clueless. Eventually, through sign language, I understood the room was $5 per night and there was no bathroom. I assumed that meant that the bathroom was shared. It did not mean that. There was indeed no bathroom, unless you counted the bare toilet bowl (no tank or seat), screened on two sides by a piece of aluminum siding and flagrantly open on the other two sides. A large drum, filled with fresh water, was provided for rinsing. The idea was that you would squat, and after you had done your business, you would locate the 50-gallon drum full of water and use a bucket to "flush". It was the same bucket and the same water you used to "shower". Completely unaware of the "flushing" protocol, I skipped this step a couple of times and eventually was given a polite demonstration by the proprietor.

The woman showed me to my room, which was behind her restaurant. Nominally a restaurant, it was really just an awning made of palm fronds, an extension of her own kitchen, where she served a traveler or two per day. As we walked to my room, the stench of rotting fish filled the air. Looking down, I surmised that we were walking through the area where she dumped her food waste, for the feral chickens to pick through. My dog, Mika, exuberantly held half a dead fish in her mouth. The reality of my situation was sinking in. I literally was giving up every bit of control over creature comforts for the sake of surfing. And it didn't bother me in the least.

I paid the woman for a week and tried to cram my nine-foot longboard into a room that was itself about nine feet by nine. I waxed up a board and headed out to catch some empty waves.

The set up was a right-hand point break. Since I am a "regular footed" surfer (meaning I surf with my left foot forward) I would be able to surf "frontside" (facing the wave) which is significantly easier than going "backside". The rip current was strong running along the breakwater. It took me almost no time to reach the breaking waves, about a third of a mile offshore. I had opted for my longboard as the waves looked small from my perspective on the beach. But I realized how wrong I had been once I reached the lineup. Rookie mistake. Waves always look smaller from the beach. I got myself in position and took off on one of the smaller sets. It closed out-- breaking all at once, leaving me no exit. I plunged into the depths and relaxed my body as I waited for the impact of the next wave to pass. Resurfacing, I reeled in my board by the leash. I was now in a bad position. Having failed to complete my last ride I was bobbing around in the "impact zone". I needed to get out of there, quickly. Especially since my board was too big to duck dive under any crashing waves. If another set approached I would have to endure its full force from the worst possible position while trying to control my board at the same time. I climbed on top of my board just in time to see another wave coming at me. This was not one of the smaller waves. This one was as tall as a house and was about to hit me with all its force. I knew there was no getting over or under this wave with my board, so I ditched the board, gulped air, and dove under. Once again, I waited for the impact to pass. When it did, still underwater, I searched for my leash to climb my way back to the surface. I found the leash and gave it a tug.

The feeling of no resistance when you pull on your leash is one of the most sickening things I've ever experienced. My heart drops into my stomach and sits there, burning in stomach juices, making me want to vomit. It is like standing naked in an open field, surrounded by snipers. You just know you are going to die, you just know it.

With nothing to pull me to the surface, I kicked my way up and gulped in air. I could see my board, bouncing in the white water, a hundred feet in front of me. There was no getting it back before the next wave would take it away. I could see another massive wave about to drill me, this time with no floatation strapped to me. I spied another boardless surfer, also white-faced and wide-eyed. The same wave had broken both our leashes. BOOM. The next wave drilled us, and the next two waves behind that one. Control? What control?

I body surfed the best I could. The rip was strong and the waves kept coming. The swim in took about twenty minutes. I have no problem swimming laps for twenty minutes in a pool, but when you have to hold your breath for fifteen seconds out of every thirty while getting ragdolled under water, it makes for a feat of athleticism. I was in survival mode. As I swam, I noticed a young Mexican man, standing on the beach with my washed-up surfboard. His eyes were fixed on me. He stood like a statue, ready to come to my aid at any moment, but giving me the dignity to save myself. His gaze gave me confidence.

Finally putting my feet down onto the sand, I saw that the gazing man was handsome and chiseled. He smiled as I approached, coughing and exhausted. He handed my board back to me and pulled out two beers from the sand, buried to keep them cool. The beers had been waiting for me to conclude my battle.

"Felicidades," Oscar congratulated me, handing me one of the beers. "Esta bien pasado hoy. Buen hecho."

He said the conditions were heavy today and that I had done well. I felt a little embarrassed, but his massive smile and rough hand on my leg as we sat sipping bears in the sand made me feel better. He invited me to join him that night for another beer at the lone bar on this island of three hundred inhabitants. I agreed.

He seemed a little drunk when we met up around sunset to

head to the bar. As we walked in, I spotted a ten-foot vinyl poster of Oscar, getting the barrel of his life. A major surf brand logo was emblazoned across the bottom left corner. My personal lifeguard was also the pride of the island. The bar was packed, and every head lifted at Oscar's entrance. Or perhaps they were looking at the tall, thick blond with him. The sound system blasted the traditional music of La Banda and people were dancing. Oscar introduced me to everyone. It was too loud to hear, and I couldn't understand anything anyway. It didn't matter. Control? What control? We headed to my Cabaña around 10 pm. I remember being drunk and very, very satisfied. After an hour we got redressed and went back to the bar. He passed me from dance partner to dance partner and, before I knew it, it was 4 am.

Something about that night I will never forget. Maybe it was getting to be a part of the local culture, or getting to be the belle of the ball with the hometown hero. Maybe it was the near- death and resurrection experience. Maybe it was giving up control completely, and being born into something new. Or maybe it was just really great sex.

Food choices were extremely limited on the island. Food rules became laughable as struggled to find something healthy to fuels myself with. Eventually, I had to give up. Each morning on the island I walked ten minutes to the only store. I bought a sope´, made of bread (yes, with gluten), beans, and queso fresco (yes, with dairy), as well as a cappuccino from the machine (yes, with corn syrup and hydrogenated oil). I would surf a few hours and then buy a snack from a kid selling something on the beach; a fried banana with caramel, sweet bread, or fruit juice. Then I'd nap, and eventually buy an unknown dish at a restaurant, do some yoga and nap some more, surf some more, buy more mystery food, and go to bed.

Day 49

After a week of staying in the fishbones cabaña, I discovered a
slight upgrade a few hundred yards up the beach. Several
other surfers were staying in the neighboring cabañas and,
once again, as the only female around, I was quite popular. I
had instant friends. There were morning surf sessions
together, afternoon story swapping, and evening bonfires
where someone would pull out a guitar, and the drunker
people would have a sing-along while the soberer of us
laughed our butts off. A few nights as I was just drifting off to
sleep a knock at the door would stir me. Oscar would come in,
fuck me hard and fast, then leave me to sleep in peace. It was
epic. The only problem with my new cabaña was that it wasn't
entirely watertight, and the rainy season was just getting
started.

I had a fitful night as the thatched roof leaked into my cabaña.
I got up twice to push my bed to avoid the drips, but it didn't
seem to help. The entire roof needed replacing. The next
morning, the waves were complete crap from the storm the
night before, but we were all chomping at the bit to surf. After
all, that's why we were there, putting up with the mosquito
bites and soggy beds. We stood in a light rain, watching the
waves, looking for anything that looked rideable. Not only
did the ocean look angry, with choppy peaks popping up all
over the place, it also looked powerful. The waves were big
and messy. My two new friends, both male, each of them a
sponsored surfer, seemed to spot something worth paddling
out for. I told them I would stay back and do yoga under a
palm tree. If I saw them get two good waves I would join
them.

What I failed to consider was that, being professional surfers,
my friends could make any conditions look fun. The waves

were breaking a long way offshore, and I kept seeing specks pop up on massive wind chops, throwing some huge aerial moves. They looked like they were having the time of their lives. After about thirty minutes, it felt like my gills were drying up. I was hungry in my bones for some waves. Or maybe I was hungry to prove I could keep up with the boys. Growing up snowboarding with my brothers, in a culture that taught women came second, I had learned to prove my worthiness by keeping up with the boys in all ways, especially athletically. I was going to go surfing! I grabbed my board and headed for the beach.

I noticed a rip flowing out next to a jetty, and assumed it would be the quickest way to get out to the break because the current would take me in the direction I wanted to go. The guys were three hundred yards to my left. I decided to let the rip take me out to the unbroken water, then paddle towards my friends in an "L" shape. When I entered the water, the wind blew spray in my face and the surface was bumpy, smacking me all over the place as I tried to stay on top of my surfboard. I looked toward my friends but couldn't see them over the surface chop. After paddling for what seemed like only a few minutes, I noticed the rip was moving me very quickly. Too quickly. I was already past the jetty, which was supposed to be to my right but now was to my left as I was being sucked away from the breaking waves and into open ocean water. In fact, I wasn't sure where I was. I sat up on my board to get my bearings. I looked to my left, and didn't see my friends, I looked to my right and didn't see the jetty, I turned around. The beach was half a mile away. I fixed my eyes on a brightly colored building on the beach. It seemed to be floating away from me, like a cloud drifting through the sky. But buildings don't drift, surfers do.

Panic seized my body. My stomach twisted, as if large hands were wringing it dry. I sat motionless on my board, but the current was still dragging me at double-digit speeds out to sea. I took a deep breath and scanned the surface texture of the water, trying to ascertain the direction in which the rip was moving. I made my best guess, based on my experience watching rip currents. I set the nose of my board perpendicular to the direction I estimated the rip and began to paddle. On that day, The Voice sounded like a middle school girl, texting her frenemy about stealing her boyfriend:

You stupid bitch. What the hell were you thinking! You are going to die. This is how it ends. Congratulations, you idiot, you just committed suicide.

My shoulders were burning, my heart rate skyrocketing and my breathing erratic. I was crying and it seemed impossible to get a deep breath or a steady stroke through my tears.

"Natasha, get a hold of yourself!" I commanded inner me. "You can panic when you get to the beach." Survival instinct shut down my tears.

One. Two. One. Two. One. Two. I counted my strokes and matched them to my breath.

Five minutes into my sprint paddle, I looked up for a moment to realize that I had made only the slightest bit of forward progress. Another wave of panic. I fought the tears again. I dug my arms deeper into the water. Fifteen minutes. Again I dared to lift my chest. I wasn't farther out, but I wasn't sure if I was closer either.

"Move toward the discomfort!" I repeated my mantra, making an effort to enjoy the burning sensation in my muscles.

Twenty minutes. I was spent, my strength and stamina were gone. Is this how my story would end?

Four years earlier
The Voice reminded me that skipping one workout was where
it all starts. It was 11:30 PM and I had just checked into my
hotel only to find the gym already closed. Everything in my
body was screaming for rest. I downed the complimentary
bottle of water in my room and felt nauseous. I thought about
making myself throw up, but I knew there was nothing in my
stomach and the nausea was from exhaustion rather than
eating. A couple of hours earlier I stood in the checkout line at
a gas station in the middle of Nowhere, Texas. I had been sent
there by my company on a last-minute trip, to deal with an
issue one of our clients was having with our product. It was
9:00 pm, and I had just traveled two time zones, having left
another hotel room in another state at 6:00 am that morning. I
was scheduled to be in another city and yet another time zone
by the next day around the same time. A bit of nodding off at
the wheel had prompted me to pull over. I held a 5-hour
energy shot, a large black coffee, a sugar-free energy drink, a
pack of sugar-free gum, a pack of beef jerky, and a Snickers
bar. I avoided eye contact with the cashier, who would surely
judge me for the chocolate bar. I handed over the money and
cracked open the energy drink. I downed the entire can in the
parking lot and ripped open the plastic on the Snickers bar. I
sat in my driver's seat, chewing slowly, crunching and rolling
the sweet goo around in my mouth. Before I swallowed I
reached for the empty energy drink can, lined up the opening
as if to drink from it, but instead spat all the calorie-laden
black sin out into the can before it had a chance to punish me
with its calories. It didn't count if you didn't actually ingest it.
I reached back for the candy bar and continued chewing and
spitting until I had devoured the rest of the bar.
I pulled out of the parking lot and continued to load my body
with enough chemicals to ensure I could make the rest of the
three-hour drive to my hotel without falling asleep at the
wheel. As I drove, I entered the beef jerky into my calorie

tracker app. Everything else was calorie-free. The tracker said
I was at 970 calories for the day and just 4 grams of
carbohydrates. I felt pretty satisfied with those numbers, but
hopeful the hotel had a gym that stayed open past 11:00 pm,
just to get in a little extra cardio.
When I finally arrived at the hotel I found the gym already
closed. So I put on my sneakers and headed for the stairwell of
the eighteen-story hotel. Somehow, I would summon the
strength to run all the stairs three times.

———

And this would be no different. Four years ago I wanted
something badly enough that I was willing to die for it. I knew
about control. I knew about mind over matter. And at that
moment Both my mind and my body wanted to live. I found
the combination more powerful than any will power I had
ever been able to summon in the past. For the first time ever, I
had want-power.

Somehow, from a place deeper than the well of physical
strength, a last burst of effort rose up. That effort felt more
painful than anything, yet I embraced the pain, letting it fuel
me.

*You will paddle until you are safe. You've done harder things for
stupider reasons. You have the strength, just summon it!* I
reminded myself I could feel any emotion I wanted, I could
give up all control, once my feet hit the sand.

By the time I broke free of the rip, someone had spotted me
with binoculars and a crowd had gathered on the jetty,
completely helpless to do anything. They watched as my feet
finally hit the sand. I stumbled onto the beach, ripped the
leash off my ankle, dramatically flung my board at the
ground, and collapsed into a heaving heap of tears. Now,
safely on firm ground, I allowed myself to experience the full

———

weight of the emotions I had held at bay. And the tears felt good.

By the time I sat down for lunch, I felt alive like never before. I ordered something I couldn't pronounce and sat back to wait. Meals in Mexican restaurants take a long time to come to the table. I was presented first with sliced cheese and tortilla chips, all of which I ate while I waited. Then, pickled spicy carrots and onions, which I also ate, until my mouth felt like it was on fire. Then my meal came, with breaded chicken, rice, salad, black beans, and six or seven tortillas on the side. The waitress set everything in front of me and then apologized, left, and came back with a side of mayo. I began slowly eating. I had never experienced such a lack of urgency to get food into my belly. I ate everything, down to the last tortilla. It was the same amount of calories that a typical binge would have been, but it was different. It took five times the amount of time to consume. It took willpower to keep eating rather than to stop. And I tasted every bite, rather than just the first two.

When the waitress returned to ask if I wanted more (like they always do), I consulted my Spanish dictionary, looking up how to say, "I ate too much." I replied, "No, estoy bien, ya comi demasiado!" (Thanks, but I've already eaten too much!) A huge smile lit up her face and she shot back "Que Bueno!" (How good!)

How good indeed.

Day 51

I sat down with the guys for a victorious post-surf breakfast of bacon, eggs, tortillas, and a cold coconut.

"Yo Nati! Mi amigo, Roberto."

One of the local guys introduced me to another local surfer.
Natasha was a hard name for many people to remember,
being so uncommon in Spanish, and "Nat" sounded funny, so
my friends started calling me Nati, and it stuck.

Roberto was in his mid-twenties, five foot five and a hundred
twenty-five pounds of pure muscle. Like most of the local
surfers, he had knotted ropes for arms and a six pack for abs.
Roberto gave me the casual Mexican handshake that young
people used, an open palm slap followed by a fist bump,
"¡Estas bien grande!" he greeted: "You are good and big!"

Big. I was big. At five foot nine, I towered above the locals. I
often hit my head on awnings when I walked around the
market. On that particular day, I had just surfed three hours
without a break, and would paddle out later that afternoon for
another four hours. The day before I had surfed eight hours
total. My back muscles looked like they belonged to one of
those bodybuilders, rubbed down with bronze goo, flexing on
a stage and forcing a smile. My butt was enormous. While my
waist might have been a size 4 or 6, my butt was a 10 or 12.
For the last six months, I had surfed an average of three to
four hours per day. A perfect day was one in which I surfed at
least two hours, did yoga, and went for a run.

I was very muscular, yes, but I wasn't all muscle. Not by any
stretch. Like an overly sheltered teenager, off to college for the
first time, my appetite rebelled in its newfound freedom. I had
been eating as much as I wanted (which was a lot!) of
anything I wanted (which included a lot of sugar and
processed foods) for weeks. I had cellulite. My legs jiggled
when I walked and my thighs rubbed together. My six pack
had turned to a soft belly. I had to buy new bathing suits
because I was popping out of all my tops. Big. Yes, indeed, I

was good and big.

Roberto reached over and pinched a thick layer of fat covering my thigh. "Come tus huevos mamacita." Eat your eggs, sexy momma. Emotions flooded in. I knew it was a compliment, but it didn't feel like one. There I sat in a bikini, no makeup, salty hair, hairy legs, eating a mountain of food, and a man was pinching my fat. Suddenly my ravenous appetite disappeared. The smile left my face and I offered the rest of my breakfast to Roberto, "Gustas un poco?" Roberto pushed my plate back to me, saying something about how I needed power to surf another three hours with him later. Then he grabbed a handful of love handles, licked his lips, and uttered the unthinkable, "Come, Gordita." Eat, *chubby* girl.

Four Years Earlier
Kurt and a friend were going to surf a very localized, hard-to-access, secret surf break. I was invited along. My heart leaped. Kurt had grown up here, but I was a transplant. By the unwritten laws of surf culture, for better or worse, you don't bring novice surfers to locally run breaks. And if you are not with a local, you don't even try to surf there without someone who is. I was in. It felt like a victory. But I was nervous. I felt like crap that day. In fact, I had been feeling a nondescript "crap" feeling for several months. At twenty-five pounds under my natural weight, I had no energy, my bones felt cold and the thought of getting off the couch made me a little nauseous. I knew surfing was way above my energy level, and that to surf while feeling the way I did was a great way to get hurt. But I hadn't yet had a workout that day, and no amount of crappy feeling was going to make me skip a workout! So, it was either surfing or high-intensity interval training. Surfing sounded a lot better.

Hoping a little sugar would pick me up, I threw an apple into my backpack along with my wetsuit, booties, and hood. Walking out the door, I second guessed myself.

A whole apple? That's like 15 grams of sugar! That's going to knock me out of fat-burning mode! I'm going to store that in my liver, which means I'm going to store water with it. I've gotta weigh in tomorrow and that's definitely going to affect my number. No way! I'll just eat half.

I took out the apple, sliced it in half, and stuck it in a ziplock. My anxiety was quieted, for the moment.

Kurt, his buddy, and I started the one-mile-plus trek to the surf spot on foot, hiking down a cliff face with nine-foot longboards, then across a beach, paddling around a point, walking across a second beach, and finally paddling another third of a mile out to the break. I was in agony before we even finished the hike down the cliff. Every cell in my body screamed for fuel. Finding none, my cells went searching for fat to burn. At the time, I was in the single digits for body fat percentage. I know because I checked weekly, carefully recording each skin fold measurement within an app on my phone. Certainly, no glucose was available for fuel, because I hadn't touched carbs in a year. And no body fat was available for fuel, either. So, my body resorted to cannibalizing its own muscle. I could feel nitric acid being dumped into my system to burn muscle for fuel. It made me nauseous. But I attributed the nausea to having eaten the apple-- well, half an apple. Guilt from 7.5 grams of sugar made me want to puke.

As we walked along the cliff, Kurt's buddy eyed me, remarking "You don't look too happy..."

More guilt. What's wrong with me? Get it together! You are being given an opportunity few people ever get!

"I'm just tired today, but I'm stoked to surf," I lied, more to myself than to him.

By the time we reached the take-off zone, I was spent, mentally, and physically. I was nauseous, and the corners of my vision were black. With each paddling stroke, my shoulders screamed for me to stop. I was shivering under my thick, 4/3 wetsuit, even though I had only been in the water for fifteen minutes. I paddled for four waves and missed each one, maybe because I was drained, but probably because I was scared. My subconscious knew that I was in no condition to survive a big wipeout, so when it came time to take the last stroke, the stroke of do-or-die commitment, I backed off.

Kurt's buddy paddled over and explained to me that the waves were softer than the beach break I was used to surfing, and that I had more time than I thought to make my pop-up. This assurance settled my subconscious, and I went full force on the next wave. I made it to my feet and for a split second felt victorious. But before I could savor the moment, my body, pushed to its limit, said enough is enough. My knees buckled, my board pitched forward and I somersaulted backward, toward the crashing white water.

Everything went black. Up became down as I spun like a sock in a dryer. A hot flash tore across my shoulder, but panic blocked the pain as I fought frantically to find my leash. I was being dragged underwater by the board, still attached to my ankle, which rode on without me. I thrashed underwater until I caught hold of the leash. My board stood upright on the surface like a tombstone, and I climbed my leash toward a second chance at life. I breached the surface, gasping for air. It wasn't until the fourth breath that I noticed blood in the water. Although I felt no pain, my fragile body heaved with sobs. *What the fuck is wrong with you, you stupid bitch?* The Voice was certain that I was an awful human being for taking such a huge wipeout. Humiliated, I let the white water push me to shore so I could calm down before going back out. The boys were still out. I should be out too.

Shivering, I picked up my board and waded to the beach to sit for a minute before mustering up the courage to try again. I examined the board, feeling relief when I saw that a fin was missing. A three-inch gash had been cut though my wetsuit and into my bicep. Pain throbbed and blood issued from my shoulder. I made the connection between the missing fin and the flash of heat I had felt as the wave expended her power on me. With a missing fin, there was no way I could continue my surf session. I was excused.

The boys continued to surf. I made the mile hike back out, dumped my board in Kurt's truck, and forced my tears to shut off. I reminded myself that shivering burns calories, as do physical and mental trauma, and walking. I proceeded to walk the additional two miles home, bleeding, shivering, exhausted, and alone.

———

I finished my eggs and promptly retired to a shaded hammock. A couple of hours later, I woke and lifted my head to see that Roberto and the guys were already back in the water. The point break was going off on that day; three hundred yards, head-high barrels were lining up. I grabbed my step up shortboard. The paddle out was brutal. The current was so strong that I had to enter a quarter of a mile farther down the beach than the point I wanted to reach. Leaving the sand, it was a sprint paddle against a river-strong current for nearly a quarter of an hour. Heavy sets were coming through. Walls of whitewash, tall as trucks, slammed me into the sand ten feet below the surface. I controlled my breathing. Inhale, stroke, exhale, stroke. One final duck dive, dipping my board skillfully under a crashing lip, and I broke free from the impact zone. A huge smile wrapped around my face, I paddled up next to the boys. A big set was stacking up and I was in the perfect spot. Roberto and the other locals were shouting at me, "Go Gordita, go!" The nickname made me laugh. I felt strong as I stroked in, popping to my feet in one catlike movement. My glutes fired as I harnessed the speed from the drop down the face. I pumped my legs, sending the board higher, to the unbroken part of the wave. I could see the lip towering over me. I threw my hand in the face of the wave to slow my speed and let the lip pitch over me, sending me completely inside her barrel. Eyes wide, heart pounding, soul on fire, I ducked just a little...I was just the right size to fit into the ocean's embrace.

After a time on the island, drama lust and addiction to the unknown appeared, like itches in the middle of my back. I agonized over the decision to stay or to go. The waves were good, the living cheap and the people amazing. But there was so much more to be explored. I called Sean, the guy I had been dating back in San Diego, to tell him how much fun I was having and how good the waves were, but also that I wanted to go explore more. He said something I've since repeated to myself many times, whenever I've had to make a difficult choice.

"Natasha, I don't think there is a wrong decision here."

While I had been traveling, we texted every day. I had the best of both worlds: my sexual freedom but also a best friend and chat partner from whom I had ample space. Sean, on the other hand, wanted a real relationship. He was lonely without a woman in his life. I brought him a great deal of happiness. It felt awful to think I might take that away from him.

Before I left, he asked me directly for how long I thought I would be gone. The truth was that I didn't know. The part of me that thought I would be gone forever was much bigger than the part of me that planned to come back. But I felt like I was choking when I tried to answer his question truthfully. I felt that old, familiar tension in my chest, but I didn't listen to it. So, instead of answering him, or admitting to myself what I really wanted, I held on to my apartment, my furniture, my kitchen items, my camping gear, my snowboarding equipment, my bikes, and my boyfriend. I lined up a friend to sublease my apartment and take care of my stuff. I lined up a manager for the yoga studio and told her I would be back in one hundred days. I lined up Sean, a man I could fall back on. When he asked when I would be back, I told him the same lie I had fed myself: in a little over three months. I was too scared of letting everyone down to admit, even to myself, what my heart really wanted.

I had been traveling for close to fifty days when I told Sean about the amazing uncrowded waves I had found on the tiny island. An avid surfer himself, Sean agreed to come visit for a few days. I left the island to go pick him up at the closest airport a couple of hours away. We spent a whirlwind long weekend holed up in a beachfront cabaña with an ocean view. He splurged, renting the nicest place on the island for $20 per night. We had a shower and a toilet that flushed. I was living in luxury. I could sit up in the morning to see waves from the front window. It was a surf couple's dream. Although I kept trying to stay on the opposite corner of the island from Oscar's house, I walked the opposite direction any time I saw him. I hoped he wouldn't see me and had assumed I had left for good when I left to pick up Sean.

On the first full day of Sean's stay, we enjoyed a post-surf breakfast at a beachfront cafe. I paid a few cents to connect for an hour to the only source of satellite WiFi on the island. Right away, my phone exploded with messages. I had been completely off the grid for a few days. Most of the messages were from my Mom, wondering if I was still alive. But one was from the woman who was subleasing my apartment back in San Diego. She said there was a gas leak and she'd needed to contact the property manager. The onsite manager already knew I was out of town and that a friend was watching my place. Although he was fine with this arrangement, the property management most definitely was not, as I would find out.

Over the next day or so, through a series of confusing emails and text messages, coming in at random times over an unreliable WiFi signal, I discovered that my tenant had been abruptly evicted. Basically, I had only a few options:

I could pay rent on a vacant apartment.

I could break the lease and forfeit both the security deposit and my belongings.

I could return home to reclaim my stuff and/or my apartment and return to San Diego life as I once knew it.

I had no means to pay rent on a vacant apartment, so that option was out. Going home to gather all my stuff from the unit, renting a storage unit, and then coming back to my road trip was also out of my budget. That left as options either going home and calling my adventure quits, or losing all my stuff.

The next morning, I felt nauseous. I hadn't been eating as much as I normally did because I felt guilty eating that much in front of Sean. I was also restricting my eating and increasing my workouts for the week leading up to Sean's visit because, although the Mexican men accepted me at my current weight, I assumed Sean would want a more SoCal look. As a result, I had lost a couple of pounds. I thought I looked great, but physically I felt awful. My body had weight loss PTSD and was freaking out, thinking I might be going back into old food restriction patterns...which I was. I was completely depleted of energy. The mere thought of paddling out that morning was making me sick. I knew I needed to rest. I sat at the open-air breakfast cafe and connected to the WiFi while I watched Sean go for his morning surf. I had a message from my former subletter, demanding I give her all her money back for the headache she endured. Another message was from the landlady, saying she needed either next month's rent or permission to enter the apartment and remove my stuff so she could get a new tenant.

I watched as Sean caught a big set wave. I turned off my phone. I ordered a fruit plate. I felt the warm sun on my face and dug my toes into the sand. I ate my fruit and then ordered eggs. I scarfed down my eggs with three tortillas before Sean finished surfing, so he wouldn't know how much I had just eaten. Then I sat and thought about nothing. I heard birds and waves. I felt full and happy.

I saw Sean catch a wave and straighten out his board, aiming for the beach. He was coming in. I knew what I had to do. I knew if I talked to him I would chicken out. I switched my phone back on, and as Sean walking up the beach toward me, board in hand, grinning from ear to ear, I sent off one text to the landlady.

This is my official notice to vacate my unit, effective immediately. Any items left behind may be removed at your discretion.

I switched the phone back off just in time for Sean to arrive at the table. He leaned in and gave me a giant kiss, dripping cool ocean water all over me.

"Best surf trip of my life!" he said, bending down for a second kiss.

"I ended my apartment lease."

"What about all your stuff?" Sean looked confused.

"I told them to take it."

Sean looked like someone had hit him. "So what does that mean? Are you still coming back to San Diego in a couple of months?" he asked.

"It means I have no plan, none. It means I'm completely making this up as I go along." Finally, I was honest. It felt good.

Step nine of the twelve-step program I followed teaches that, if we are truly honest with ourselves and others, we will "know a new freedom and a new happiness...We will comprehend the word serenity and we will know peace...Our whole attitude and outlook upon life will change. Fear of...economic insecurity will leave us. We will suddenly realize that God is doing for us what we could not do for ourselves."

And, in that planless moment, I had new freedom.

Chapter 24: No Fucks Left to Give

Day 55-69

As much as I enjoyed having Sean with me on my adventure, I was ready after four days to be back on my own. Although Sean was easy to get along with, and we genuinely enjoyed each other's company, there were two issues.

First, I had become accustomed to doing whatever I wanted, whenever I wanted. In theory, I could enjoy that freedom while Sean was with me, but I still hadn't learned how to tell anyone else what I wanted, guilty that it might inconvenience them. The second issue was something that I couldn't admit to myself at the time: when I was with Sean, all the guys ignored me. It felt like only one person saw me, but I needed the whole world to see me. I simply liked it better when I had a meaningful relationship with Sean over the phone, but also received all the male attention I could handle, right in front of me.

I drove Sean from the island back to the airport, two hours away, so he could return to California while I continued my solo Mexican journey. Suddenly, the truck lost power. I was going uphill. It was the hottest part of the day. The engine cut out. We were an hour from anything. Without power steering, I muscled the truck to the shoulder and we waited as the engine cooled. I tried to turn the engine over and got nothing, not even a click. Just a moment before, I'd been so ready to get rid of Sean, but was suddenly so grateful to have him with me. An incredible sense of guilt came over me. He suggested that I hitchhike to go find a mechanic while he waited with the truck, the dog, and surf gear.

You moron! The Voice began. *What would you have done if Sean wasn't here to watch your stuff?! You can't do this alone! You are addicted to shallow, meaningless attention, you stupid slut.*

I waved down a passing car and eventually found a mechanic. I paid the mechanic to return with me to Sean and the dead truck. Of course, when he arrived the truck started just fine, as dead automobiles do when mechanics are present. We were able to drive the rest of the way into the town of Puerto Escondido. The truck died a few times along the way, but started again each time after cooling. We managed to coast into a mechanic shop late that Friday afternoon. Of course, the mechanic wouldn't look at the truck until Monday.

Sean took a cab to the airport, and I took my boards, my puppy, and a backpack full of bikinis into Zicatela, the beach neighborhood of Puerto Escondido. Zicatela was better known as the Mexican Pipeline. I found a hostel where I could put up my hammock for a few days. The hostel was right on the beach. For a few dollars per day, I could simply lift my head to check the waves when I woke. The moment Sean was gone, my heart ached to have him back. I was so alone and helpless. With no transportation, my adventure was on hold. With no apartment back home, I was free-falling without a parachute. The Voice wouldn't leave me alone. *You're making the stupidest decision of your life. You're completely delusional to think you can do this on your own.*

I phoned Sean as soon as I knew he would be off the plane back in San Diego. I told him how much I missed him. I told him I was so nervous about the truck and about money and about no longer having a backup plan in San Diego. In true "Sean form", he was nothing but supportive. He told me to enjoy this setback as part of the adventure. He told me I could stay with him for as long as I needed *when* I returned to San

Diego. He told me I was doing the right thing.

On Monday, I tried to call the mechanic but couldn't get a good connection on my American phone. When I finally did get a hold of someone, the only thing I understood was, "Mañana", tomorrow. This fruitless process repeated itself on Tuesday and Wednesday. From what I could understand, the mechanic's secretary was telling me that I needed a different mechanic, one who worked with electrical problems. But I really couldn't pick up much of what she said.

After five days, I realized that nothing was going to happen with my truck unless I made it happen. I knew I needed help with Spanish, so I walked into town and looked around for people I recognized from surfing who might be able to help me. After wandering around for an hour, I saw one guy who spoke English and I asked him for help. He looked me up and down. He licked his lips and said he could help me if I helped him. I felt sick to my stomach and, even worse, helpless. There was no Yelp, no Google business listings, no Yellow Pages. For that matter, there weren't even addresses. In Mexico, business is based on relationships. There is just the guy who knows a guy who can bring you to that guy. But I didn't know any of these guys. I was alone.

Puerto Escondido is a surf Mecca. Puerto, as they call it, is a show. The waves are massive and most consider it the heaviest (most dangerous) beach break in the world. Kurt had traveled to Puerto on a surf trip while we were married and hadn't surfed because the conditions were too extreme. Puerto draws backpackers and those seeking a simpler life from all over the world. The air is filled with excitement from the heavy waves and the men are filled with ego from surfing those waves. It is quite a spectacle. The main road runs the length of the beach and the waves break very close to the shore. This gives even more incentive for hot-shot surfers to strut their stuff.

I was getting really anxious. There were only two places to surf in Puerto Escondido. Besides the expert level beach break, there was only one other place to surf in Puerto which was insanely crowded. I tried surfing at the crowded place and damaged my board when a beginner hit me on the first attempt. On the second attempt, I cut myself badly on a rock, trying to avoid the other surfers. On the third attempt, I got no waves at all. So I quit surfing.

Truckless, surfless, voiceless, alone, and trapped, I started to get depressed. After several days, I met a guy in a restaurant. The guy said he had a friend, Manuel, who did towing and who could help me move my truck to a different mechanic. He told me his friend spoke English. I sent Manuel a WhatsApp, and we made plans to meet at the useless mechanic's shop in the morning. I took a cab to the shop but realized that, in my panic of dropping off the truck, coasting in on a prayer, I had forgotten exactly where the mechanic was located. Not only that, but I had given Manuel incorrect information about where to meet me. To make matters worse, my phone wasn't getting any coverage in that area.

The cab driver dropped me off in a place I knew I was relatively close to the shop. Walking down the dirt path along the side of the road, I jumped as pitbulls lurched at me from behind barbed wire fences, men whistling, and calling out "Güera" (white girl) from the second story of concrete buildings. My skin crawled. A green truck that looked like it had been hit on all four sides drove by slowly, the driver craning his neck to eye me as he passed. I saw brake lights and then reverse lights as the truck backed toward me. Adrenaline pumped through my already stiff body. I pulled back my shoulders, sucked in air, looked straight ahead, and started taking longer strides.

"Nati?" The driver called at me.

Apparently, there weren't too many other big blond white girls walking around the neighborhood that day, so Manuel was able to recognize me, even at 35 mph.

"Manuel! Gracias a Dios!"

Manuel and I found the shop where my dead truck languished. Unfortunately, Manuel's English turned out to be no better than my Spanish. Manuel and the mechanic spoke for a few moments, and Manuel informed me that we would need to go to another mechanic, a few miles away. We dropped off the truck at the new mechanic, who said to call him the next day. Manuel drove me back to my campsite on the beach. In typical Mexican fashion, the mechanic's "next day" turned into several next days. Each day, communicating with the mechanic was difficult, at best. Friends from the hostel helped me with the phone calls, but still, I couldn't understand what was taking so long.

After another three days, I felt more hopeless than ever. The surf was too crowded and too scary, and I was trapped without my truck. I went back to the shop by cab to pick up my truck, broken or not. Once again, I hadn't made a great mental note of where we had left the truck, and I wandered around for an hour, under a beating, 95 degree afternoon sun, in sweltering humidity. I stopped twice at corner stores, pounding water and asking for directions, but no one seemed to know what I was talking about. When I tried to call the shop number, my phone wouldn't work.

Finally, I walked by a house, in front of which a man rested in a hammock in the front yard. I called out to him, telling him that I was lost and that my phone wasn't working. He invited me into the yard. Because everything in Mexico is relational, no exchanges ever occur without some initial chitchat in a hammock. The man gestured for me to sit in his spare hammock for a while, and I did my best to make conversation. Then, he took the mechanic's number from me and called on his own phone. In two minutes, the mechanic came to pick me up at the kind stranger's house. Another crisis solved by the kindness of a strange man.

Solved, except that two days later the mechanic told me he couldn't find the problem and that I should try to find someone else. He knew a guy, but he was busy and wouldn't be able to get to it for another week or so...*or so?*

Puerto has an infamous nightlife scene that kicks off around midnight and goes until sunrise, seven days per week. Guys with egos the size of the waves they just rode emerge at night to look for women. And the women are there, just waiting for the privilege of getting fucked hard by a guy strong enough to ride one of those waves. Since I had nothing better to do, I decided to go looking for some excitement one night.

I went out at 1:00 am, looked around the bar, and found the one I wanted. Before I knew it, he was taking me to a pay-by-the-hour hotel complete with a heart-shaped bed. He tried to get me to pay, but I had only brought enough money for the cab ride home. I clearly remember telling him, no, you can't put that in there, but oops! Oh well, I thought, at least he was small enough that it didn't hurt. So I let him do what I had clearly told him not to do. Because, well, boundaries.

After an hour was up, I stumbled out into the street alone, with no cell phone and only 40 pesos ($2 USD) in my pocket. I realized I had forgotten the name of my hostel. Somehow I pieced it together as I laughed my way home.

Yet another day passed, and yet another guy--this time, one I met at a surf shop--told me he knew a guy who was the best (no, truly, this one was the best), and that he would meet me at 2:00 pm and take me to the mechanic on his moped. Two o'clock rolled around, and surf-shop-guy didn't show up. At 3:30, I was still waiting on the steps of the surf shop when another young man noticed me. He told me he had seen me out surfing. We started to chat, entirely in Spanish. I told him why I was waiting, and he said he could help me. *Of course, he could.* He knew a guy who was the best in town and he would take me there right now on his motorcycle. *Of course, he did.* At least that's what I hoped he said; I was really only about 60% sure, but what other options did I have? Desperate, in flip-flops and shorts and with no helmet, I jumped on the back of a crotch rocket, behind a man I had met four minutes ago. I was completely and utterly helpless. I felt totally out of control. And I was starting to like it.

I giggled with terror and glee as the motorcycle guy whipped around turns showing off all the way to the shop. I followed him in my truck to the fourth mechanic shop. Once again, I was told to call tomorrow. After a few tomorrows, the mechanic informed me that he also couldn't diagnose the problem.

A few evenings later, stressed and anxious about not having a car, much money, or surf, I found myself out on the hunt again. I remember a strange feeling coming over me. It wasn't that I felt bad for what I was doing, but I didn't feel good about it either. It felt like drinking a second cup of coffee because I couldn't stay awake at mid-day, as if I was covering up a problem that might need to be addressed. Instead of being curious about the feeling, I ignored it. Back at the same club, I noticed the same surfer guy from the lovers' motel the previous week. A massive smile came over both our faces. Game on. After an hour of dancing, we left together. This time, as soon as we exited the noisy club he began speaking to me in English. I found this strange, since he hadn't appeared to speak any English on our last encounter. But whatever. Even stranger was when he brought me to his home rather than to a motel. Why hadn't he brought me here last week? And then the strangest thing of all happened. He took off his pants to reveal what seemed to have tripled in size since last week. I laughed so hard, and he thought I was laughing at him. Wrong guy, oops.

This process of failed attempts to find a mechanic able to diagnose the problem with my car repeated itself one more time, with another ride, with another strange man I had only just met and with whom I couldn't communicate well. To another mechanic shop, the fifth, where I was informed that I should check back tomorrow. That particular "tomorrow" was the day I met Diego.

Day 70

 Diego was gorgeous. Like most Mexican surfer dudes, he was chiseled. His shoulders bulged and his abs rippled. His skin was the most incredible shade of maroon. But his smile...oh, that smile. It took up his whole face. His voice was raspy and so sexy.

I met Diego while surfing, on the day that the fifth mechanic failed to help me. Having no other options, I was trying to make the best of surfing the insanely crowded point break. Diego paddled over and greeted me in Spanish. Ears full of water, I struggled to respond intelligently, so he switched to English. We chatted about the conditions that day and for how long I was in town. After a few minutes, he caught a wave and threw a ridiculous aerial maneuver at the end, trying to impress me. I caught the next wave and danced lightly to the nose of my longboard, stuck my toes over, and cross-stepped back, equally trying to impress. It worked.

We got out of the water together and headed to the cantina. He bought a coconut for me and a Corona for himself. We sat on the beach, talking Spanglish for the next three hours. I told him I wanted to go for a run and he said he would wait right there for me. Sixty minutes later, he was still on the beach, waiting for me. I told him I wanted to practice yoga and he said he would wait right there for me. After another hour, he was still there, waiting for me. Then I told him I was hungry and he took me to dinner.

Not having my truck, stuck in a place where the surfing wasn't ideal, I felt helpless and alone. Diego offered to help me find the right mechanic. And, like the five guys before him, I took him up on his offer. If I ever wanted to get my truck fixed, there really weren't any other options.

After a couple of tries, Diego and I did manage to locate the right mechanic, one who could actually help me. But something was strange about our interactions with the mechanic. Mechanico Sanchez would speak in Spanish to Diego for a few minutes. Diego would then turn to me and say "He's going to fix it. Let's go." Only he said it in Spanish. In fact, in front of other men, Diego refused to use English with me. I asked him to explain what the mechanic had said, but he wouldn't. He simply told me it was taken care of. As soon as we got in the cab to leave, he informed me that those guys knew him, and they feared him. He said my car would be fixed, quickly. But that's all he told me and would not elaborate further. Diego had it under control. I could relax. Or, at least, that is what I tried to do.

For the next three weeks, Diego never left my side for any

time longer than an hour.

I phoned Sean. In three minutes, we were over.

Diego and I picked up my Honda. I handed over way more money than it should have been but I knew I was not in a position to argue. Then, with a working vehicle, Diego asked me if I wanted to see the real Mexico. The real Mexico? I had no idea what that meant but I knew my answer was a definite yes.

Chapter 25: Off the Grid

Day 70-75

Diego was born and raised in the state of Oaxaca. He had spent his entire life surfing secret locations around the region. In southern Oaxaca there are at least twelve pointbreaks. All with sand bottoms, long rides, barrels and rippable walls. A couple of the points are well known to surfers and often see massive crowds. But many of them are accessible only by four-wheel drive or boat, and even then you better have a local with you or you will get lost or ambushed. Rumors of guys hunting down waves using Google Earth only to end up with their tires slashed, their windows broken and their camera gear stolen were not uncommon. You didn't just go to Southern Oaxaca and surf the secret pointbreaks. It was the wild wild west of the surfing frontier. You either paid big money for a guide (and still took massive risks) or you stuck to the crowded spots. Diego had been a sponsored surfer and was now a local surf guide. He knew all the locals, was friends with the cartels, and was familiar with every nook and cranny of the coast. With my car fixed, he and I took off on an epic surfing whirlwind, hours upon hours, surfing perfect waves with no one around. Or snoozing, cuddled up in a hammock in the shade between sessions. We bought fish off of locals and made ceviche daily. If we were not sleep surfing or eating we had our other favorite activity to keep us busy, at least a couple of times daily. This is the stuff of surfers' dreams. Many will pay thousands of dollars for the opportunity to drive up a hidden stretch of sand to see a perfect, barreling wave, no other people for miles. Many others are never able to find such perfection at all. I had hit the jackpot. I was getting to do it all, and in the company of an incredibly handsome and sweet pro-surfer/Latin lover, one who gushed with affection for me as only a Latino can do. I could never have dreamed of anything more.

Diego took me to meet his family. They lived in a tiny village, in a cinder block house with no windows or AC. They had no flush toilet or kitchen. Diego was the second youngest of twelve children, every one of whom had been raised in that house. I met his mother as she cooked tortillas over a stone oven, heated by a fire. His elderly father struggled out of a hammock to greet me with a kiss on the cheek. He took me by the shoulders and stepped back for a better look. I was at least four inches taller than him and outweighed him by a great deal.
"Dame un niñeto." A huge grin lit his face as he asked me to give him a grandchild. I could see Diego's smile within that grin.

We stayed a couple of days in Diego's village. A decent beach break layout front, completely unknown to white people. As I'd observed in other small Mexican communities, a complete and utter lack of stress coexisted with extreme poverty, and a sense of total contentment prevailed. Families passed the hot days together, hanging out in their open-air homes, laying in hammocks, and chatting with neighbors. During the cooler hours, people took on small amounts of work, such as basic farming, fishing, harvesting fruit, and cooking. Some families earned a tiny amount of money by operating small stores from which they sold a couple of bottles of water or a few packages of chips per day. As much as they were businesses, the stores were places for families to hang out together. The cashier might be nine years old. Seated on woven chairs in front of the store, you might find teenage girls passing their babies among one another.

Families might also draw income from small restaurants,

which functioned like the stores, as places to kick back with those closest to you. Occasionally a few pesos were earned. Huge smiles seemed to be a requirement for living in Diego's village. Earning an income was not. It became clear to me that, for some on this Earth, life was not a struggle. There was a second way. Family, friends, relationships, and community.

Day 76

Diego told me of another secret location, even farther south, and said he'd take me there. We drove on the highway for an hour, and for another hour down a washed-out dirt road. I kept asking him if he was sure we were going the right way. The road was nearly impassable. I was grateful for my four-wheel drive. Eventually, we came over a hill to see the ocean, spread gloriously in front of us--but no waves. Diego assured me we weren't "there" yet. The road ended in sand, and Diego hopped out without explanation. He circled the truck, letting about a third of the air out of each tire. He got back in and simply pointed down the beach. I put the truck in the lowest gear and carefully rolled onto the soft sand. The truck slowed and the RPMs shot up, but all four tires gripped and we started to make our way across the beach. What looked like a steep drop lay about a mile ahead, and I grew increasingly nervous as we approached it. The closer I got, the more I could see. I realized we were at the top of a large sand dune.

"Do we have to go down the hill?" I asked, assuming that if we went down we might struggle to get back up.

"Mamacita, no te preocupes. Tengo muchos amigos por acá, pueden ayudar, todo bien, tranquila."

Upon his admonishment, I quit worrying and kept driving as instructed. As we crested the dune, two things quickly became apparent. First, a perfect barreling wave--with absolutely no one around--awaited us at the bottom of the hill. Second, the hill was probably way too steep to drive back up. But the allure the wave eclipsed any need for control as I plowed through the sand down the steep incline.

The wave was perfect, too perfect. We were exhausted after only an hour from having ridden so many waves. We were also starving and parched. The mid-day sun beat down, and no man-made made structure was visible in any direction. I always kept extra water in my car, but I knew three liters would hardly get us through the day. And there were also the problems of food and shade. When I mentioned these to Diego, he scowled and asked why I never trusted him. He told me to put my board under the car, grab my water and a hat, and follow him. I obeyed.

We hiked for fifteen minutes into the jungle down a narrow, machete-cut path. The path took a turn, heading straight up a mountain. After another ten minutes, the jungle canopy parted to reveal a small hut with bamboo sides and a palm frond roof. A little trickle of smoke snaked from a hole in the roof. Diego whistled loudly. A man ducked to exit the hut and emerged, hunched, shirtless, and skinny. He appeared to be about two hundred years old and waved at us vigorously.

Facundo was a dive fisherman. He lived for his entire adult life in the hut he had built on a cliff. He owned the land on which he'd built the hut. In addition, he owned a few sets of clothing that hung from a line inside the hut, reeking of campfire smoke. He had a hammock and a few improvised fishing tools for harpooning fish and hooking octopus. Other than those few essential items, Facundo owned nothing at all. His smile lacked several teeth, but he didn't need them as he sat on a rock, slurping oysters right out of the shell. He hacked one open and handed it to me. It was the size of my hand. I had tried oysters a couple of times at a fancy restaurant, but only with lots of lime, hot sauce, and horseradish. But Facundo's oysters were huge and impossible to swallow whole, so you had to chew their mushy flesh. I gagged and nearly threw up as I tried to slurp it down. He saw I was struggling to eat it, so he hacked me open a second shell, scooped out the flesh, and rinsed it in some murky water stored from a hacked-off two-liter bottle. He handed me the brown and white oyster, presenting it on a dirty hand alongside an already squeezed slice of lime. The second oyster, anointed with a single drop of lime juice, was no better than the first. I politely refused a third, saying I was already full. Facundo dug into another hacked-off plastic bottle, extracting three small octopuses from its turbid waters. Proudly, he mounted one on each finger, holding them aloft with a huge, toothless grin and crying "Foto, foto!" as he handed me his flip phone. The octopus was then sliced, doused in lime juice, and handed to me in chunks. This second course was a significant improvement of the first, and I ate until I was truly satisfied.

After we had eaten the equivalent of about 100 American dollars' worth of seafood, Facundo led us on a tour of his land. He guided us to a mound of oyster shells; there must have been at least ten thousand. Then, Diego and Facundo disappeared into the palapa without inviting me in. I eavesdropped from outside. Surprisingly, I understood quite a bit of their conversation. They were conducting a business negotiation. Apparently, Facundo had asked on a previous visit for Diego to find a buyer for his property. Diego had indeed found a buyer. The asking price was 1.5 million American dollars. But I could hear the older man growing heated. He demanded, "Where can I live where people will not bother me? I like being alone, I like it here on the mountain with no one else. Where will I dive? I don't want to eat and get fat like people from the city. "

 It was amazing. This man had absolutely no idea what $1.5 million would do for him for the rest of his life. But he didn't care. Money had absolutely no value to him. He preferred to eat octopus and sleep in a hammock, in filthy clothes, all to preserve his lifestyle. I was amazed. This man had found a second way...a way that was starting to resonate with me.

Diego and I stayed a couple of days, surfing until the swell dropped off. We cooked over a campfire and slept on the beach under a million, trillion stars. We ate fresh fish, caught by handline, and drew fresh water from Facundo's well.

Finally, it was time for an actual bed and a shower, so we said goodbye and packed the truck. I had been dreading this moment from the time we drove down the dune.

As I had anticipated on the ride down the steep dune, we did indeed get stuck on the drive back up its severe slope. I hit the gas, and the wheels dug deeper. Diego screamed for me to stop. I obeyed. I had some 2x4's, cut at a hardware store in San Diego, just in case this situation ever materialized. We dug the boards into the sand under the tires. Diego pushed while I drove. We made it out of the hole and returned to the base of the hill. We let more air out of the tires and tried again. Once again, the truck sunk into the soft sand, and once again we dug it out. Diego's face whitened. I started to get pissed, more at myself for trusting him than at him for getting me into this mess. After a third, exhausting attempt I was livid. As Diego pushed the truck out of the hole for the third time and the tires caught, I drove away from him at full speed back down the hill. I whipped the truck around on the flat sand and got a three hundred yard running start. I was driving way faster than I felt comfortable with, and the back end of the truck fishtailed violently. I hit the dune at a gentle angle and floored the gas pedal. I whizzed by Diego, who stood dumbstruck at the crazy lady behind the wheel.

 It worked. I nearly caught air as I crested the dune. Diego was still down on the beach, holding two blocks of wood, but I wasn't stopping until I hit hard-packed dirt. I reached a dirt road a couple of kilometers away. I parked the car in the shade, let my dog out to play, rolled down the windows, reclined my seat, and closed my eyes. An hour later, Diego appeared, sweating and huffing. He woke me from my nap and we both had a good laugh.

Diego and I spent the next two weeks adventure surfing through the region, living off of pennies, sleeping anywhere the surf was good, and having the time of our lives. It was like something out of a romance novel. But the plot would take a dangerous twist.

Chapter 26: Red Flags

Day 80-86

For a brief second a pulse of anxiety shot through my sternum. I was gathering dirty laundry from the truck. A Spanish version of the Big Book of Alcoholics Anonymous peeked out of Diego's backpack. I took a deep breath, reminding myself not to have "boyfriend in recovery PTSD". I brushed it off, hoping it was just something from his past.

Diego didn't like to speak to me in English, which left me guessing a lot. It also put him in a position of power. He knew the area, the roads, the locals, the places to sleep, the places to find food...without him, I would have traveled only to the spots in my travel guide book or those I found from Google reviews. With him, I was on the adventure of a lifetime! I was surfing unknown breaks and venturing to places other California surfers would pay thousands to see.

But he wouldn't ever give me any details. Possibly that was because he didn't have any to give. I never knew where we were going, why we were going there, how long we would stay, how we would eat, or where we would sleep. I don't think he did either. Sometimes he would wait until 11:00 pm before answering my questions about where we would find a place to sleep. He didn't have a care in the world, and since I wanted to continue scoring epic waves and epic hammock time, I was forced to release control and go with the flow.

It was the rainy season and the bugs were awful. My body was covered with infected insect bites. Some nights we got a room with screens, out of the rain and away from the bugs, but other days we got wet. I was surrendering control for the sake of surfing, adventure, and romance. Surrender was new and exciting, and it was giving me a high.

One day, when we were running low on gas, I mentioned to Diego that I wanted to drive a few miles in the wrong direction to fill up before heading out to seek the day's waves. My personal rule was never to let the gas dip below half a tank. He told me no, that we had plenty, and said there was another gas station in the correct direction. I asked how far but he didn't answer me.

When we arrived at the service station, almost on empty, we were told, "No hay," or "There is no gas today." Diego fired a couple of questions I didn't understand at the gas station attendant. Then he looked at me and commanded, "Lets go, fast!" I had learned to do as I was told. I drove, and I drove fast. After a few minutes, we caught up to a pickup truck with large racks extending from the bed. There was a huge tank in the back, maybe five hundred gallons of liquid sloshing around inside. Diego ordered me to flash my lights and honk. I obeyed. He took off his sunglasses and hat and stuck his head out the window to be recognized. The truck pulled over and three men jumped out, all wearing bandanas over their faces. Diego told me to stay put and I didn't argue. He got out of my truck, casually strolled over to the men, and greeted each of them with a hand slap and a fist bump. My heart was racing. He returned to me and stuck his head in the driver's side window.

"Dame quinientos pesos." He asked for 25 bucks. I gave it to him. One of the bandana guys sucked on a hose, spit gas from his mouth, and filled a small container. He brought the container to my car and told me to unlock the gas tank. I obeyed. A full-service filled up from the cartel, which had just robbed the gas station ten minutes before. I wondered if I should leave a tip.

"How did you know those guys?" I asked Diego as they drove away.

"I know them." He responded.

A few nights later, in a tiny fishing village of about a thousand people, I decided to treat us to a decent dinner. There was a pizza parlor in the village, and I was sick of fresh fish tacos. Diego, who just last week seemed to have an unlimited supply of money, was now out, completely out. He told me there would be more money soon, and would I just pay for the food and the cabana rentals this week, and that he would pay me back. I was running out of money too, but what was I supposed to do, leave a man to starve? My "out of money" and his "out of money" were very different. I still had a few grand in a savings account, credit cards, and parents. Diego literally did not have a dime to his name, but he didn't seem to be too worried about it. I was finding so much value leaving worry, stress, and control behind that I decided to just go with it.

I stuffed my mouth with pizza, enjoying the grease running down my chin, and heard a commotion outside the restaurant. Several loud trucks had rolled in, and I heard Diego's nickname being called out. Diego told me to stay inside. I obeyed. Although I could hear the conversation outside, I couldn't understand it. Too many voices were speaking at once and I couldn't make sense of the Spanish. But the other people inside the restaurant did understand, and all were staring at the empty chair next to me where Diego had been sitting. The conversation got loud and heated. Eventually, the trucks fired back up and peeled out. Gravel sprayed audibly against the side of the building as the trucks spun their tires.

Diego returned, looking sad. "I need to get out of this state. I don't want to kill the people." And that would be all he would say of the incident. He ordered another beer, his fifth, or maybe seventh, I had lost track. Then he ordered a shot of mezcal, "for his nerves", finished it, and ordered another. I would have no explanation, but I would have a large bar tab to pay.

After a while, he was drinking every day. A lot. He was drunk most afternoons by three or four. As the drinking continued throughout each day, his personality changed. He started verbally abusing me by seven or eight in the evenings: I smelled bad, I needed to shave, I was a slut, he just knew I was off with other men while he surfed, I didn't love him, I only cared about money, I was racist, I thought I was better than him. On and on it went; the more drunk he became, the more hurtful his comments. But the next morning, it would be all, "Princesa, te quiero." (I love you, Princess). That, or his favorite, "Let's make a cappuccino baby, you bring the milk, I'll bring the coffee." Every morning, I would tell him it was over if he ever spoke to me that way again. He would cry and say he didn't remember it and he was so sorry. He probably didn't remember, and he probably was sorry, but within two or three days the story would repeat itself.

But Diego had run out of money. I was running low myself but his out of money and my out of money looked different. I had a savings account in case I wanted to return home and pay the first month's rent and a security deposit on a place to live. I had a car. I had parents with money and credit cards. Diego could not afford to eat. What was I supposed to do? Leave a man to starve. But he showed no signs of wanting to earn money. Part of this was due to the fact that he was happy to sleep in a hammock and live off fish and part of it was that I was treating us to dinners at restaurants and buying snacks to have in the car whenever we needed them.

Eventually, I grew tired of roughing it every night, being eaten alive by bugs, never having a real shower, no escape from the relentless sun, peeing in the dirt, and living off ceviche. The surfing was indeed epic and my skills in the water were improving greatly. But I was reaching my limit of roughing it. I needed to find a way to earn some money and I needed a proper bed to sleep in. I had rented a cheap apartment from a friend of Diego's. The apartment was back in Puerto Escondido, a three-hour drive from where we had been surfing. It had been a long exhausting day and all I wanted to do was to get back to the apartment, fall into bed, and sleep. There was no question as to whether or not Diego was going to stay on the ranch with his family or come with me to stay in the apartment. He assumed he would come with me.

I wanted to break it off and tell him he couldn't come. I got a choking feeling in my chest, and couldn't say what I really wanted to say. It was so hard to say anything politely in my basic Spanish and I didn't have the courage to bluntly assert, "You are an alcoholic and are using me and I don't want anything to do with you anymore." I tried in Spanish to say something like he was a wonderful person and I enjoyed spending time with him but I would prefer to be on my own from here on out. But even if my Spanish was good, it had no effect on him. He promised, like he had done four or five times already, that there would be no more drinking (after tomorrow) and that he would be able to find work back in Puerto Escondido. The good little girl inside me, who never wanted to upset anyone, quit arguing and hoped for the best.

We got in the truck to make the drive to my apartment, but he directed me to drive in the opposite direction. He needed to run a quick errand in the next village over. Then we could be on our way. I was annoyed, but I obeyed. We arrived in the village--which was twenty miles out of the way--only to learn that the man he was looking for wasn't home, but would be home "ahorita" - in a bit. In Mexico, ahorita can mean anything from a couple of minutes to several hours from now. We waited, and waited, and waited. I felt simultaneously impatient and guilty for getting impatient. After all, wasn't I in Mexico to learn to slow down, stress less, give up control, and be more present? So I played soccer with little kids in the street while he drank beer. The sunset and still, we waited. Finally, I told him we had to go, that I was going with or without him. He told me not to worry, that he would drive and I could sleep and that it was better to drive at night anyway. Then he bought another beer from the corner store, and two more for his friends, and turned his conversation back to them.

Principles from my Al-Anon program started to play in my head. *You agreed to take him here, you can't blame anyone but yourself.* And, *No one has the power to make you angry except yourself.*

We continued to wait well past dark, and finally, I said what I had been wanting to say for hours, in the tone of voice I had been wanting to say it.

"I am exhausted. I am starving. I've done all that you asked, and you are sitting here getting drunk while I feel like crap. Let's go, now! Do you need me to repeat that in Spanish for all your friends to hear?"

I turned my back to him and walked to the truck. I fired it up and put it in reverse. He was quickly in the passenger seat. By that time, it was long past dark and my eyes were beginning to feel heavy. Diego kept begging me to let him drive. Even though he was twenty-nine years old, I had reason to believe he had probably not driven more than a dozen times in his life. On top of that, he had been drinking all day. I was clearly frustrated with him, and the more I complained of being tired, the more he insisted that I let him drive. The roads seemed to be getting narrower and narrower as we wound along a mountain road, hugging the coastline. A huge storm the day before had washed rocks down the steep mountain, rocks that now filled the already narrow shoulder to my right.

As we rounded a sharp bend, I had to slam the breaks when a truck appeared in my lane less than thirty feet ahead, coming straight at me. The rain had washed huge piles of rock and dirt into the truck's proper lane, so the driver had swerved into my lane to avoid them. Thirty minutes later, I was the one swerving into oncoming traffic when my headlights swept around a curve to reveal that the road was completely gone in front of me, washed out, leaving in its place a gaping hole and a sixty-foot drop down the sheer side of a cliff.

"You are going to kill us, mommie!" Diego shouted at me. "Let me drive, I'm from here. I know these roads!"

"FINE!" I caved in, wanting to trust him.

I pulled over at the next turnout and we switched seats. He adjusted the mirrors and the seat, and we buckled up as he slowly pulled out. Diego maintained a death grip on the wheel, hands at two and ten o'clock, as we proceeded very slowly and in complete silence. He was driving well under the speed limit, and it seemed like he was swerving slightly. But I was so tired, I considered that maybe I was just imagining things. A two-ton truck behind us started to tailgate us, flashing his lights, but Diego continued to drive exquisitely slowly. The truck honked, prompting from Diego, "Why are they gonna be in such a hurry to die? I got my baby in the car. I don't have hurry!"

I wanted to mention that sometimes it can be more dangerous
to drive too slowly, and that we were hardly moving, but I
kept my mouth shut. The truck found a break in the curves
and passed us on a straightaway. It was going on 1:00 am and
I hadn't really slept at all the night before which we had spent
using our surfboard bags in the sand as a bed. I closed my
eyes and tried to sleep, ignoring his bad driving, convincing
myself that everything would be fine.

Another truck, this one a semi-truck towing a huge load,
became annoyed with our slow progress along the treacherous
road and began to tailgate. The rumble from the diesel engine
woke me when the truck downshifted and punched the gas.
The driver was about to pass us, going uphill, around a curve.
I sat up in my seat just in time to spot a pile of dirt and rock
spilling into our lane from where it entirely covered the
shoulder. The truck was neck and neck with us on a road so
narrow that two compact cars would have a hard time driving
side by side. As the truck passed, Diego swerved to avoid the
rocks, edging just slightly to the left.

The awful sound of smashing metal still rings in my ears. The
front driver's side quarter panel of my Honda SUV crumpled
like playdough, no match for the semi-truck. The back of my
Honda fishtailed to the left. I had a clear view of the front end
of my beloved truck heading straight for the mountain on the
right. Diego gripped the wheel and corrected. I screamed as
the passenger side mirror smashed into the mountain, sparing
the rest of the truck by just inches. The semi-truck continued
on its merry way.

We pulled over as soon as we were able and switched seats.
Diego was happy to give over the wheel, but wasn't about to
surrender control. He began a tirade about how the driver had
tried to kill us, had tried to kill ME, the person he loved. Diego

was furious with the driver for swerving into our lane, endangering me. I mentioned that Diego himself had kinda sorta maybe swerved a little bit too, but Diego reminded me that I had been sleeping and hadn't seen it, so how would I know. I agreed and shut up. He insisted we find a 24-hour liquor store so he could get a shot of mezcal to calm his nerves. There was way too much Al-Anon going on in my head at that moment for me to agree to that request. So, just as Diego liked to do, I simply did not respond, even after the fourth demand. I did however cave in when he told me I must overtake the truck, get far enough ahead that I could stop into a police station and notify the authorities that I had been hit, claiming I was the driver, and ask them to please come out to the road and stop the truck. However, when I did so, the policy laughed and said they would "look out for the truck" without ever getting up from their card game.

Diego stayed with me for the next several days. Although I refused to buy him alcohol, he was more or less drunk the entire time. But he never had money when it came to mealtime. I felt so bad when he would tell me he was hungry. Principles from Al-Anon resounded in my mind as loudly as the crunching metal of my truck. Each time I got in my car, I had to forcefully yank the door open because the collision jammed it. It opened with the worst nails-on-a-chalkboard sound you've ever heard, but all I could hear was the Al-Anon detachment flyer: *Our role is not to prevent a crisis if it is in the natural course of events.* What I didn't know is just how rapidly the crisis would present itself.

Day 89

A few days later, Diego was to give an afternoon surf lesson, and announced that he was going to treat me to dinner with his earnings. Evening approached and I made my preparations. I shaved my legs, found a dress tucked into the bottom of a backpack somewhere, and even dug around in my toiletry bag for lip gloss and eyeliner. My face hadn't seen makeup in a month. I took my time getting ready, waiting for him to come home. It got dark. The lesson would definitely be over by then, so I texted him. No response. I called him. No answer. I was getting hungry, so I made a snack. An hour later, I made another snack. After a further hour of waiting, I put on my PJ's and started a movie on my laptop, so much for date night. I fell asleep alone.

One year earlier

It had been six weeks since Kurt had relapsed for the first time in almost seven years. Maybe his relapse was just a slip and would soon be a thing of the past. Two weeks before his relapse, when Kurt said I was too fat for him to be sexually attracted to me, I had asserted that if he didn't start treating me with respect, I would leave. Then, when he relapsed, I reluctantly gave him thirty more days to prove it was just a slip. If it was more than a slip, I would leave, just as he had told me to do when we were dating:

 "If I ever relapse, promise me you will leave me. It won't be quick and it won't be easy."

Six weeks after the relapse, I was still with him. He appeared to be clean, but he also hadn't changed. He was aggressive, blaming me for not appreciating him when he financially supported me, giving me the opportunity to pursue my dreams. He wasn't interested in sex, or working more than half a day, or conversation (unless it was to pass judgment on his friends, claiming his program of recovery was much better than theirs). He wasn't interested in getting off the couch, for that matter. I would later find out that he had been lying to me about his sobriety for those six weeks. But I was still new at living with an active addict, so I didn't catch it.

I was surprised when I came home to a dark house one evening, after a late night at the yoga studio. I felt a little relief that I didn't have to walk on eggshells while I prepared my dinner and a little more relief that I wouldn't have to ignore the TV while I ate, while Kurt ignored me and watched his shows. After I had showered, eaten, and cleaned up dinner, I was ready for bed but he still wasn't home. I texted him a message.

Hey, did you go to a meeting or something?

No response. My first thoughts shot up from the worst place, but I reined them in. I grabbed a bowl of ice cream, since he wasn't there to judge me for eating it when he already thought I was a fatty. For a few moments, I drowned my anxiety in sweet cold cream. After another hour, I decided to call. Straight to voicemail.

I grabbed the laptop and typed in "Find My iPhone". Heart pounding, I entered Kurt's iTunes password--which I had memorized. The system was unable to locate the phone. It had been turned off or had a dead battery.

I sent one more text.

Please, if you get this, can you please just let me know you are okay? Come home whenever but please just let me know you are alive. I love you.

After forty-eight hours, he finally texted to let me know he felt miserable and had been up for two days straight.

Ditto, I texted back.

—

I had been sleeping for several hours when I awoke to pounding on the door. I flipped on the lights and opened the door to face a strange man. The man was worked up, speaking quickly, and I couldn't understand what he was telling me. Asking him to slow down, I was able to make out the words "Diego" and "jail" and "money". My Al-Anon programming kicked in full blast, and I absolutely refused. No way in hell was I going to bail Diego's little ass out of jail! The man explained to me that Diego had told him where some money was stashed and asked me to go retrieve it. I went looking and, sure enough, I found six American twenty-dollar bills, enough money to buy food for 3 weeks for both of us. *You little bastard!* I thought as I handed over the money. The strange man left, and I went back to sleep. But my night wasn't over.

A couple of hours later, I awoke again, this time to hear Diego fumbling with the lock. I got up to let him in. He looked like hell and smelled worse. When I demanded an explanation, he started crying. He caved and admitted to me that he was employed as a personal bodyguard to a member of the Mexican Cartel. They had been drinking together that afternoon and, from what I could understand, they had crashed their car into a liquor store while driving drunk. The police were nearby at the time of the incident and, when they tried to arrest the man whom Diego was sworn to protect, Diego did his job. He disarmed the nearest cop, gained control of the cop's assault rifle, and with the weapon pointed at the cop's head, he ordered the rest of the officers to drop their weapons and get on the ground. The scuffle continued for several minutes until the national guard showed up, and Diego was forced to surrender. Both Diego and his protectee went to jail and were released hours later with a $60 USD fine. Friends in high places.

I said nothing while he told his story, my mind replaying images from Mexican movies we had watched together, about cartel girlfriends getting kidnapped and held for ransom. Part of me still wonders if Diego had made it up, trying to sound more important than he was. I wasn't really in danger, was I? I remembered the look on one kind Al-Anon woman's face, when she told me, *Be sure you leave him when he's not home.* I had brushed off her warning.

As soon as I could tell he was passed out, I packed my things in the dark. By 6:00 am, my truck was loaded and I was on my way to find a new place to call home. But something was different. I wasn't scared. I wasn't mad. I was laughing. The Voice told me that I was a total idiot, and making all the same mistakes again.

Yup, I was. *This shit is too funny.* This time it took me only a month to see that what I had gotten myself into was making me smaller. Last time it had taken over a year. I counted my relationship with Diego a success even as I kissed it goodbye. I turned up my tunes and drove into the sunrise to find a fresh start. I had no idea that I would soon be actively searching out even more dangerous situations.

Chapter 27: Where oh Death is Your Sting

Day 91

I had returned to a somewhat known point break where I could live cheaply. I was hoping to perhaps do beachside massage on traveling surfers to earn enough to keep going as well as to hide from Diego. I rented a unit in a three-story adobe home. The house was about a five- minute drive from the waves, tucked away in a quiet corner of a tiny fishing village. There I could be alone with my hurting heart. I needed some time to mourn the loss of Diego, which felt like losing Kurt all over again. I knew it was over, I knew he was all wrong for me, but I wished it could have been different. I made a run to town for supplies and wasn't planning on leaving the village for a few weeks if I could help it. For the first two days, I surfed and cried for hours. I slept like a rock in my comfy bed. But the third night would be nothing like the first two. That night I will never forget. If marked a new era in my life.

On the third night, I fell asleep while writing melancholy poems in my journal. As there was nothing to do after dark it couldn't have been later than 9 pm by the time I was old cold. And then it happened.

The television fell from the wall, piercing midnight silence to shatter into a million little pieces. Dishes crashed. The entire, three-story adobe house shook violently. I tried to get out of bed, but it was impossible to stay on my feet in the pitching room. I crawled to the floor and made my way on hands and knees to the middle of the room, settling in a spot between two supporting pillars. I was on the second floor. Getting down the spiral staircase was impossible due to the rolling floor. It seemed like ocean waves were lifting and lowering the floor at least three feet up and down every couple of seconds. I was trapped inside. The shaking got worse, and cracks ripped audibly through the concrete walls upstairs. Loud as a freight train, the earthquake picked up speed. At the epicenter, less than 30 miles away, clashing tectonic plates ramped the magnitude to 8.1. The house was old. The notion of building codes or structural inspections applying to this tiny Mexican fishing village was laughable. The power grid went out, and midnight darkness fell entirely into pitch blackness. The awful noise of everything breaking continued.

At first, I was only a little scared. I had been through earthquakes before, and was certain it would stop after a few seconds. It didn't. The floor pitched so violently that I couldn't stay in one place. I heard masonry grinding upstairs, bricks coming loose. The earthquake roared on, gaining momentum, and seconds stretched into days. Eventually, I realized that this earthquake was the Big One, and knew I was going to die.

I placed one hand on either pillar. Suddenly, I was five years old again, in Mrs. Meyer's Sunday school class. I was wearing my blue cotton dress with big white buttons, and patent leather shoes over thick white tights. Seated at a preschool-height table in the basement of an old church building, I was coloring a picture of a Bible story. In the picture, a man with long hair and big muscles pushed against two pillars while the building around crashed.

The story goes, God had given this man, Samson, Hulk-like strength. Samson used the strength to destroy members of the enemy tribe. The author worded the story like this:

Then Samson reached out to the two central pillars that held up the building and pushed against them, one with his right arm, the other

I stood in the adobe house, one hand on either pillar. Surrounded by deafening noise, certain that these were the final seconds of my life, the five-year-old within me had not a care in the world. She colored contentedly, at peace. The scene played out like climactic, slow-motion images from an action movie. Fire burns an entire city. Skyscrapers collapse. In the middle of the apocalypse, there stands the hero, stoic and unmoving.

I heard the story above me start to cave in. At that moment, completely accepting things I could not control, I was alive like never before.

I am going to die, and that is really okay. It's been a wonderful ride. I lived a full life. I'm happy to move on now. Goodbye struggle, goodbye pain, goodbye control.

I have never known such serenity.

And then, just like that, it was over.

I later discovered that the third story was completely destroyed, and that the entire building was moments from collapsing in on me.

Immediately following the earthquake I took some locals in my car to check the ocean for signs of a tsunami. We tried driving up the mountain to higher ground but the roads were too dangerous, filled with boulders and gaping holes. The journey could not be made in the dark. I spent the rest of the night in a hammock outside my house avoiding the aftershocks which might certainly destroy the house

---

completely. I'm not sure I slept at all. The next morning presented several issues. First, I needed to call my mom, ASAP. International news of an 8.1 earthquake with an epicenter just 30 miles from me certainly would have made its way back home. But in my new-found boldness, I had ventured far from the beaten path. There was no cell service in the fishing village. Also, we were under a tsunami warning. Anyone in the village who had someplace else to go had already evacuated. Finally, there was no water in the village. The purification plant had been damaged. I remembered a place I had surfed with my ex-boyfriend, maybe twenty miles away, with a high cliff to which you could drive. The cliff jutted out into the ocean and seemed like my best option for getting a cell signal. And it would provide higher ground for protection from the possible tsunami.

Staying in the village wasn't an option. Trying to navigate roads that largely had fallen into the sea took a couple of hours. Eventually, I found the spot and was able to send a text to my petrified mother.

With the roads so dangerous, and my rented home destroyed, I was completely stranded on the deserted cliff. Now that I was safe from rising waters, there was nowhere else to go. The precipice overlooked a perfectly breaking, right-hand point break wave with no one on it. Control? I couldn't care less.

I had with me half a raw chicken on ice, purchased the previous day. It would go bad if I didn't cook and eat it soon. I had five gallons of water, a few tortillas, some leftover veggies, and a handful of fruits. I was completely unprepared for camping. There were no houses, no restaurants, no man-made structures at all, nothing. I was perched on a desert cliff at the edge of the sea.

 After a couple of hours on the cliff, I spotted two local

fishermen coming in for the afternoon. I approached them to chat and offered to share my chicken with them. I was going to cook it on a stick over a fire, since I had no dishes. The men agreed to help me cook, and said they could track down some kitchen gear. One of them left, assuring me that he would return. An hour later, he emerged from the jungle, accompanied by three more hungry fishermen. They carried a big pot, some mismatched plastic bowls, and two spoons retrieved from their fishing shack two miles down the beach. With a huge smile, one man flashed me his missing teeth and said "Vamos a hacer un caldo de pollo" or, "We are going to make a chicken soup." He made a great show of the announcement, as if we were about to eat steak and lobster. I dug in the car, finding a coffee mug and a blender pitcher to add to the cookware. An hour later, we had all eaten until we were full, and there were enough leftovers for breakfast the next morning. I still have no idea how half a chicken fed six of us. I was reminded of another Sunday school Bible story coloring page: Jesus with Pantene Pro-V hair, Clorox-white robe, and blue sash holds a small basket containing three fishes and a crust of bread. The story goes, Jesus used the food in the basket to feed five thousand people, with thirteen baskets of leftover food.

Over the next several days, I discovered that I had guardian angels, ones who fished and conspicuously lacked many teeth. I was completely out of food and water, but you'd never have known it. The fishermen brought me coconuts to drink, massive catfish they had speared, oysters the size of my hand, reptile eggs, and fresh octopus. They fetched me freshwater from their well and carried it in a bucket on their shoulders two miles. They cooked something different for me every night, and there was always enough left over for a meal in the morning. They strung up a hammock thirty yards from my spot, stationing at least one of their group to watch over me, twenty-four hours a day, to be sure I was safe.

I was in heaven. I was sure of it. I surfed each day, alone but for the turtles. The surfing was super fun. It was consistently head-high and offered rides up to a hundred yards. At night, I'd never seen so many stars. In much of Mexico, the mountains drop sharply into the ocean, making for waves much faster and heavier than those found on shallower, gently sloping coastlines. This geography meant I was literally surrounded by mountains and ocean. For hours each night, I saw lightning strikes over the mountains, but no rain ever interrupted my sleep under numberless stars. Surfing twice a day, I did yoga on the cliff and napped in the shade. For eight days.

So close to nature, eating only natural foods, waking with the sun, having only the light of a fire at night, being in the ocean for hours, and having absolutely no control over anything...I have never felt so connected to a power greater than myself. One day, running on the empty beach, I heard someone call "Nali", my Mexican nickname. I stopped and turned, searching a full 360 degrees. There was no one, nothing for miles. But I heard what I heard.

Much later, it struck me that I had undergone a time-tested awakening experience. Almost all spiritual traditions include a narrative in which the spiritual pilgrim journeys alone into the wilderness, and there undergoes a profound spiritual encounter. I felt something inside me had died, and something new was growing in its place.

To paraphrase Mark Twain, I was no longer afraid to die, because I was no longer afraid to live.
I couldn't control a single thing, even if I had wanted to, and was utterly at peace.

I had gone through hell with my marriage, my body, and my

finances, and I had survived.

I had been stripped bare of everything--no food, no roof over my head, only the items in my car. And yet I was fully provided for and, might I say, happier than ever.

There was nothing to accomplish, nothing to produce, achieve or become. There was no need to control how I spent my time. None of that would get me anything I really needed since I already had everything right there on that cliff.

There was no one to impress with my body, no one to judge me for my food choices.

There was no Mom, who might find out what kinds of naughty things I was doing. I had no need to control my desires.

Eventually, my body had to return to civilization. I was covered in mosquito bites and had grown leg hair like a wolf. Every tiny scratch on my body festered, infected with what would turn out to be staph. My flesh was being eaten away by salt water, and sand fleas fed on my open wounds. I had been using a surfboard bag as a sleeping pad, and a smaller board sock for a sleeping bag. The arrangement was less than ideal. I had been out of fresh water for days and drank only from coconuts. I had lost several pounds and was dying for some green veggies. I needed medical attention and a bed.

At last, word came that the roads were now cleared of boulders and repaired after the earthquake. I was exhausted. I needed civilization.

Day 100

When I received a reasonable offer for my yoga studio in San Diego, my desires registered loud and clear. I didn't have to think twice. I left my perfect waves and cliffside home, found an internet cafe, printed, signed, scanned, and emailed the paperwork back to the broker. And, just like that, my life in San Diego was over. I bought a plane ticket home to train the new owner and to get rid of any remaining items I had in storage. But I left my truck, my puppy, and my surfboards in Mexico with a friend. I was certain that I was coming back.

After two days in San Diego, I had completely lost my voice. My voice was how I got what I wanted. I was very good with my words. But in Mexico, with the language barrier, and all the time I was spending solo, I hadn't spoken much at all in three months. I had gotten used to going with the flow, rather than arguing for my way. After four days in San Diego, I had the flu, completely run down from the stress of reinhabiting my old life. After ten days of weight scales and full-length mirrors, access to salads, and SoCal botoxed women everywhere, I regressed into restrictive eating behaviors. I felt like a big fat cow. After two weeks in San Diego, I couldn't wait to get back to the simple life, nothing to prove, no one to impress, no goals or accomplishments to pursue. All I wanted to do was to be. My days of trying to prove myself were over.

I had arrived, I had made it, The Voice assured me. I was going back to Mexico. From here on out, life would be perfect.

So, after quitting my entire stateside life, I returned to the Mexican Pipeline, Puerto Escondido. I paid upfront for five months of rent on a small apartment and got a job teaching yoga and doing massage in a spa that catered to tourists. The pay wasn't great but I could make enough to cover my room and board. There was nothing left to control. I bore no more worries about body fat percentages. I had plenty of attention from men. A had two or three guys at a time whom a simple text would summon if I was feeling in the mood. When we finished, they would leave me alone without complicating my life. I could eat whatever I wanted, surf as much as I wanted, stay out dancing with boys as late as I wanted. There was nothing left to struggle against, no drama. Nothing was left to accomplish, achieve, produce or become. At last, I could quit trying to prove anything to anybody. I could just be present, living a simple, Mexican seaside life.

Every problem I had been fighting to control had vanished. Now I had a new problem: there were no problems. Life was perfect. Way too perfect. I became completely depressed and overrun with anxiety.

Chapter 28: Getting Big

"So whenever a person becomes too interested and eager to calm down the mind, he creates many problems for himself." -Osho

When Kurt and I were newly married, he'd received an invitation to stay with a friend in Puerto Escondido. The stay happened to be over my birthday. He asked if I cared, and I said I didn't. I lied. But it was a surf trip and, being a surfer myself, I understood. When Kurt returned from Puerto Escondido, he had no gift for me, no souvenir, nor had he surfed Mexican Pipeline. He hadn't felt comfortable approaching the Pipeline, opting to surf some other, safer locations. Kurt was a very good surfer. He was my surf mentor. He had been surfing for over thirty years. He knew his limits. And now, I woke each morning to see those same, expert-level waves, breaking just a hundred yards from my front porch.

Zicatela Beach in Puerto Escondido is nicknamed "Mexican Pipeline" for a reason. The waves behave similarly to those of the "Banzi Pipeline" on the North Shore of Oahu. I wanted to surf there, but had yet to do so. I wasn't convinced I could.

At the Mexican Pipeline, the ocean slopes up steeply, or the land falls away quickly, whichever way you want to look at it. This slope creates a shelf beneath the surface of the water. Storms formed in the South Pacific travel from south to north across the globe. Having gathered steam in their travels, the storms hit this underwater shelf at Zicatela with astonishing force. The waves jack up in size and break top-to-bottom, the lips of the waves pitching forward to create hollow tubes. A surfer can attempt to wedge herself inside of such tubes. The dangers of attempting this maneuver are numerous and severe.

First, if you don't paddle fast enough, and don't get to your feet fast enough, the lip will pitch you over the top. Surfers call this "going over the falls." The name is apt, which any surfer knows when she has experienced the weight of a waterfall drilling her to the ocean floor.

Next, if you do happen to catch the wave and get to your feet at the exact right time, and manage to get yourself into the barrel, then you have to worry about getting yourself out of it. Too much weight on the back foot, and you are dragged up the face of the wave, once again to be spit "over the falls". Too much weight on the front foot, and you nosedive. You must generate enough speed so that, when the barrel reaches its finish, you come out before the lip closes briny curtains on you. But you want to stay in as long as possible, because...well, because it feels better than sex.

Getting barreled is like union with the divine. Imagine a lover so glorious, so massive, so infinitely more powerful than you. The lover allows all of you, your entire being, to come inside and experience her greatness for just a second or two. She permits your entrance only if you are good enough, respectful enough, gentle enough, strong enough, practiced enough, and completely willing to abandon any attempt to dominate. She requires you to harmonize yourself with her own motion. And, even then, it is completely up to her whether you enter, and whether you get to leave alive. *That* is getting barreled.

Of course, there are further dangers after you finish a wave. There are always more waves just behind. Each one waits to smash you as you attempt to get back to the spot where you started.

Now, take all of those dangers, turn the dial up to 11, and you have a big day at Zicatela. The waves, already notorious for being more powerful than any other place on earth, present faces that reach sixty feet. Imagine a wipeout at Zicatela like being pushed off the high dive only to have several pools dumped on top of you. If you do manage to surface there are more pools tipping out over you just as you suck down a breath or two. Repeat this process for each wave of the set, up to ten or twelve times, and eventually you find yourself washed up on the beach thanking your stars that you made it out alive.

So there I was, on the pacific coast of Mexico. No real home, no possessions, no decent job, no boyfriend, no plan. The last time I felt so free I was 16, considering where my life would lead me. But to be honest, I didn't feel free at all, not when I was 16 and not then either. What I felt was anxious.

What will I do about money? This question started to take up a lot of space in my brain. I had had enough to get by but I wanted security. My conditioned mind said not only did I need to worry about financial security, but also I needed to be doing something worthwhile with my life. I longed for purpose. My anxiety wasn't quieted by a small weekly paycheck. Just like when I was 16, worried thoughts about what I would do to derive my purpose and meaning in life plagued me. Those familiar words were still haunting me. "You are special." "You are going to do something great one day!" "You can do anything you set your mind to." But all I was doing was teaching yoga to a few worn-out surfers, earning enough to meet my most basic needs.

In the absence of major life problems, drama, and big projects, a deep and penetrating anxiety bubbled up from my depths. The anxiety certainly had been there all along. It was what kept me running from one task to the next. I stayed busy to avoid feeling it. Now with waves, I was scared to surf and nothing to distract me, the stillness became overwhelming. *Oh my god, I am nobody! No one will ever know my name. I'm screwing this all up. I have just this one shot at life and I'm not doing anything significant with it.* I would lay in my tiny Mexican studio during the hot afternoons, after a yoga class in the morning and before an evening of massage work. Anxiety would shoot through my chest, as if I had drunk too much coffee. I tried reading and watching Netflix, but the anxiety was too strong. I needed to achieve something.

The problem organizing your life around overcoming problems is that, as soon as you overcome them, you go looking for new ones. If life is about accomplishment and achievement, then you are bound never to achieve the greatest accomplishment of all: peace. And so it was with me.

The anxiety masqueraded as hunger. There was no good reason for me to be hungry right after a meal, but I was. As soon as I was bored, I was hungry. If I was shopping for food, preparing food or eating food, I felt much better. I recognized the anxiety-driven hunger for what it was, but that didn't make the hunger go away. I allowed myself to give into it when it became too overwhelming, consuming bowl after bowl of cereal and milk. Sometimes meditation helped but mostly was either working on something, eating something, or being eaten by anxiety.

My heart has always told me that I was put on this earth to help women. I thought I could fight my anxiety by coming up with a plan that accomplished three things: it helped women, it paid my bills and it allowed a schedule flexible enough to surf every day and to travel. There was a fourth item on the list that never made it consciously to the surface. But my ego was very clear that whatever this thing was, I was going to look good in front of a lot of people doing it.

I realized my new struggle: Surf Mexican Pipeline, look good

doing it, build a social media following and use it to earn
money and help people.

A thousand reasons not to try it flooded my mind. What if I
break my board or my leash and get held down without
flotation? What if the lip lands on my back or my knee and I
get injured? There were risks, very real risks. I wasn't afraid,
but I had massive respect for the power of those waves. Every
morning for a few weeks, I took my camera and a mug of
coffee to the beach, talking to surfers as they entered and
exited the water. I photographed the waves and studied the
surfers' movements. I made mental notes about where they
paddled out and how they handled being caught in the impact
zone after a wipeout. One day, I left my camera at home,
taking a pair of fins instead. It was a "small" day, but I could
tell it was more powerful than anything I had ever
experienced in the water. And I was going to enter without a
surfboard, without a giant floatation device strapped to my
ankle.

I spotted a group of surfers I knew. I swam to them so as not
to be alone. Arriving at the group, I explained that I was
testing the speed and power of the wave, getting to know it. I
felt a little more confident knowing they were going to be
watching for me. A set came through, and I dove deep to
avoid it. The final wave of the set was the biggest, and I was in
a bad position. I dove as deep as I could, but it was shallow.
My belly scraped the sand, just a few feet deeper than the
crashing lip. I was unable to avoid the most tumultuous part
of the wave. I completely surrendered to the washing machine
effect and, several seconds later, was released on the other
side of the wave, gasping for air, drained of energy, but alive
like never before.

The swell lingered over the next couple of days, and I body
surfed six or eight powerful waves. With no board and no

popping up to my feet, I was able to experience the feeling of hurdling myself over the ledge with no risk of getting impaled by my board or dragged underwater by my leash. My confidence grew.

I waited for the next "small" day, finally paddling out on a surfboard, I sat where the waves seemed smallest. It took several minutes of all-out battle just to get past the breaking whitewater. It took an additional hour to catch two waves. I fell on the first, but was thrilled with myself for having even attempted it. The second wave barreled, and I felt a rush of victory just before it smashed me inside. I clearly remember surfacing for a breath and saying to myself, "Oh my gosh, I *can* surf this place!"

I continued to surf for the next several weeks, any time the waves were small. My wave count was improving and so was my confidence. Each session felt like a triumph when it was over, but felt like a war zone while I was in it. I glanced constantly at my watch, hoping two hours had passed so I could call it a day. Every second stretched my comfort zone. I was so loaded with adrenaline that it exhausted me.

When the waves got too big for my skill level, I would peer through my camera to watch the better surfers. They pulled into barrels big enough to hold a house. It was almost a relief when the swell outsized my skills. When people asked me if I had surfed that day, I could respond, "Oh, no way, too big for me!" It was nice to have an excuse not to go out. I knew I had to respect my limits. But my heart told me I could do anything I wanted to do. And my ego wanted to go big. Never in my life had *intermediate* been acceptable. I was either the ugliest in the room or winner of the beauty contest. The little girl inside of me who had been told that women were created to submit to men wanted so badly to join the men out there on the battlefield...just to prove she could.

On one of the extra-large days, I sat on the beach, watching the pros paddle out. It was so big that specialized equipment was necessary for survival. The pros used huge, pointy boards called "guns". They wore floatation suits that made them look like sumo wrestlers. They had special leashes, made extra thick with quick-release pins just in case they went "over the falls" and their board dragged them underwater. These men were going to war. They were athletes of the first class. Their minds and bodies were prepared for the battlefield. I was at the beach early because the force of the waves was shaking my apartment and woke me before dawn.

When the ocean has that much energy, the entire town does as well. The surf paparazzi already gathered on the beach. Drones equipped with cameras filled the sky, a buzzing, voyeuristic flock. I laid out my towel and snapped a larger lens onto my camera. Looking through the zoom, I spied a pink surfboard in the lineup. *That's funny.* In big wave surfing, the pros like to use colorful boards so they show up better in photos. Apparently, some guy wanted to stand out badly enough that he surrendered to the idea of a pink board. A few minutes later, the pink board and its rider took off on a massive barreling wave. The surfer looked like a rock climber on the edge of a massive sheer cliff. Snap snap snap, I shot about twenty frames. I touched the camera's display screen, hitting the zoom button to admire the wave.

"What?!"

I said it out loud, even though no one was close enough to hear me. I was shocked. The pink-boarded surfer was a woman. I looked back to the other surfers in the lineup. I looked back down at my camera. I looked up at the sky. *Holy crap! Women can do that too!*

I drew a quick breath. Anxiety fired in my sternum. *If that woman can do that, why can't I?* A dare had been dangled before me, and my ego wouldn't let me say no. The anxiety spread, threatening to crush my lungs. She was the only woman out there, doing something most men would never dare to do. I knew there were only a handful of women who could even come close to riding waves like that. I knew I could be one of the best in the world if I tried, that I could do "anything I set my mind to". And I wanted it, badly. I wanted the adrenaline, the risk, and the danger. I wanted to stand at the edge of human experience and then leap off. I wanted to do something extraordinary. I was empowered...and terrified. Suddenly, I knew my next challenge. I would surf big waves.

The plan was simple. Become a big wave surfer, get amazing photos from surfing big waves, post them to my social media, gain a big following, become an influencer, use my influence to help empower women and earn a paycheck. It ticked all the boxes. I would earn a living, surf as much as I wanted, help women, and of course gain the validation I still so desperately craved.
I don't remember another time in life when I've been so sure about anything and so bound and determined to make it happen. I was a pro at mind over matter. I could self-discipline better than anyone. I could take a beating. I could put in the work. I could and would become a big wave surfer.

I studied the waves at Zicatela for days before getting in with swim fins, just feeling the power. Eventually, I took a board out on a small day and caught a couple of heavy waves. I felt like I had just won the lotto. After that first wave, I clearly remember kicking out and thinking to myself, "I *can* surf these waves!" Game on!

One does not just become a big wave surfer overnight. I was still very much a novice surfer. There was much to do! The rule of 10,000 says that to become an expert at anything you must spend about 10,000 hours doing it. I calculated that would mean training eight hours a day for the next five years. Waves are rarely surfable for more than four hours per day due to tides, winds, and swells. That meant I would need to spend multiple hours training in other ways. Big wave surfers need to be exceptionally strong to survive life-threatening conditions. They need to have incredible breath-holding ability. They need excellent surfing technique, because even tiny mistakes can be fatal. And they need to be fearless.

In addition to surfing as many hours as possible daily, I began my training in other areas. I started a brutal dryland training routine involving hours of high-intensity intervals, sprints in the sand, and going to the gym daily. When my body was so exhausted that it refused to move, or when I was recovering from one of the many injuries I sustained while taking my chances in bigger and bigger surf, I would study surfing videos. After taking a class designed for big wave surfers, I began training in free diving and breath-holding.

I became addicted to the feeling of being without oxygen. It is a euphoria, only experienced when one pushes past the limits of what seems humanly possible. Everything goes numb. You lift out of your body. Your mind goes to a still place. You want to give up, your body convulses, but your mind pays no heed. In this state, you learn who is boss. You learn that your mind can and will override your body if you train it. Ah yes, the familiar old control high.

I was feeling that high the first time I forced myself to blackout. It felt like refusing food when I was starving. It felt like stepping on the scale and seeing a lower number. It felt like putting on clothes that had become too big on me.

When I'm about halfway into a maximum length breath-hold,

my lungs start to feel panicked and desperate. My body fights for survival. But my brain knows better. My brain has a lot of practice in controlling my body. My brain understands that I'm only halfway there, and even if I push a little too hard, the worst-case scenario is that I black out. In which case, I'll involuntarily resume breathing with no long term negative consequence. The body will always have the last word.

As I pushed toward my first maximum hold, the convulsions continued and strengthened. I told myself to feel and enjoy them. I told myself that it is just a sensation. I told myself to move into the sensation. I recalled an old mantra I used to tell myself: *Hunger is the feeling of being skinny.* This was just another uncomfortable feeling. For a second, I noticed that my extremities were numb. My heart had stopped pumping blood to them in order to preserve blood flow for vital life functions. I liked this feeling. I told myself to like this feeling.

I told myself to move into the fear, to feel it, to make friends with it. At some point, I realized: *I am not going to stop. I am not going to draw another breath.* I felt utterly at peace with this. The sensation in my lungs was awful. My legs felt like I had been sitting on them for hours, but my mind was blank--no, better than blank. My mind was high. Convulsions shook my entire body. Every fiber of my being screamed for breath, but my mind was getting a control high.

I felt so proud of myself for being able to deny my needs that I actually loved the feeling of being without.

I felt the blackout approaching before it actually hit. There was a moment in which I chose to move toward it rather than away from it. I tapped my stopwatch to end the count. Feeling my body slipping away, I embraced the fear of what might come next. I have no idea for how long I was out, but my guess is only a few seconds. When I came back, the first thing I noticed was a vibration. The entire universe was vibrating. My ears were ringing and my surroundings were in black and white. Slowly, the ringing stopped, color returned and the vibrations around me stilled. But my body still buzzed. It seemed like minutes elapsed before I was even aware that I could move again. As soon as I could, I looked at my stopwatch. Five minutes and three seconds had passed between breaths.

Another part of my training focused on overriding my body's natural response to fear. Ask any big wave surfer if they get scared and their response will be, "Yes, that's why I do it." The idea is not to become fearless, as that would be impossible, but to feel the fear and move toward it. Any normal person naturally backs away upon sensing a dangerous situation. But backing away from a wave at the wrong time can be deadly.

When you are taking a wave, there is a moment in which you must commit 100%. There is a point of no return. If you are not beyond certain that you are going to ride this wave, then you will do something to prevent yourself from going for it. Sometimes, as much as I wanted to, my body refused to do the deed. I would paddle as hard as I could but at the moment I needed to jump to my feet, I would sink the back of my board and back down. In big wave surfing, the consequences of this minute pause can be fatal. If the surfer backs off just a split second too late, the wave picks her up and throws her over the lip into the worst possible position. The hapless surfer enters "The Impact Zone", where waves crash like bombs. And even if you do pull off early, the rest of the line up gets pissed at you for wasting a wave. You have to contend with more waves, behind the one you just wasted, approaching to devour you.

I would get so angry at my body for having the final say. I was going to teach it who was boss. My mind would find a way to override my body. I had no idea I was doing what I had already been practicing for years.

I decided to go hunting for fear, any place I could find it. To muster courage in situations with big consequences for messing up, I felt I most certainly needed to master myself in matters of little consequence.

I was a squeamish eater. I hated fish; it grossed me out. I once threw up after taking a big bite of clam chowder which I mistook for corn chowder. The truth is that I feared fish.

I had already encountered "pescado entero" or whole fish. A fish, fried in oil, with nothing but the guts removed, served on a plate with the head and tail still intact. I was shocked when a head appeared on my plate, eyeballs gazing up at me in silent accusation. I was further shocked when I later discovered that the head, brain, and eyeballs were considered the best part of the fish, traditionally reserved for the head of the household.

"Just eat it. Eat one eye. What's it going to hurt?" The guy at my table pushed the fish head toward me.

"No way! I've had enough to eat. What's it going to get me?" I retorted.

He replied simply. "Balls."

He had a point. I used my fingers to scoop out an eye. I chewed exactly once. It didn't pop as much as I expected it to. But neither did I. Something clicked. If I wanted to do scary stuff that could kill me, I needed mental strength. Over the next few weeks, pig brains, bovine testicles, raw reptile eggs, and live grasshoppers would become part of my big wave training program.

Crunching on grasshoppers or holding my breath until I passed out was one thing. Getting pitched over the lip of a wave as big as a house with enough force to break my back was another. But surfers did it, all the time. It was doable and I knew it. People take wipeouts, big, gnarly, heavy wipeouts, and they survive them without injury. I knew what I had to do, I had to take some of those wipeouts.

It all started innocently enough, the slipping-back into control mode, the attention-seeking, the living from ego rather than authentic desire. Surfing, which was once the only thing getting me out of bed in the morning, became the new means by which I would force my body to earn the approval I still desperately craved.

Part III - Sex

Chapter 29: Money is the Easy Part

Money was constantly on my mind. I wasn't going to become a big wave surfing with 50,000 Instagram followers overnight. I had hatched the perfect plan. But what was I going to do while I executed it? Anxiety weighed heavily on me as I watched my remaining savings drop dangerously low.

I needed to make a trip back to San Diego, where I still had health insurance, to have my annual cancer screenings. I was scheduled to be there a week, crashing with my friend, Brooke. On the first night of my stay, I started telling her about my financial worries.

"Listen," she said, "I have an idea. Maybe you could stay here in San Diego a little longer and work. I need a roommate this month because I can't cover the rent on my own. And you need to make some money."

Right away, I knew where this was going. Brooke was also a massage therapist...but not the kind of massage therapist I was. I knew Brooke for two years before she told me about her line of work. I always wondered how she never seemed to work but always paid her bills. One day, she explained to me that she did sensual massage. I thought that was kind of cool. I was married at the time, but I wished I had that kind of freedom. She said it made her feel empowered. She said she loved it.

"If you want to make some good money, you could just work out of my house for the month," she offered.

The idea scared the shit out of me and turned me on at the same time. Brooke gave me the details. I'd have to be topless, wearing just my panties. I'd have to let guys touch me. And

I'd have to touch them, everywhere. The amount of money I could make in one day would cover my living expenses for a couple of weeks. It sounded fun, sexy, and risky--all the things I loved! But me? What if someone found out? What if they knew what Natasha from the town council and Natasha the owner of the yoga studio was really doing? And could I really do that? I mean, it felt wrong. What if these men were married and being dishonest with their wives? What if the police showed up? And what if, god forbid, my parents found out? I was breaking so many rules. It felt...sinful. Sinful and oh so sexy!

If I was going to become a big wave surfer, there was no way I could train the number of hours I needed, travel around the world to the best waves, and work a normal job. This was the perfect solution. I estimated I could earn enough in a month to live for six months in Mexico. I would only need to do this a couple of months out of the year. I would still be working toward my real goals for empowering women and surfing big waves. This was just a temporary means to end, I told myself. I agreed to stay with Brooke and give it a shot. I changed my return ticket so that I could stay for a month.

Brooke showed me which websites to post on. Together we picked an alias for me. I chose "Katie" since I had a friend in high school by that name who always had been the kind of sexy I wished I could be. Brooke took photos of me in lingerie for the websites. Nervously, I hit submit. Brooke told me to get my makeup and hair done because the calls would start coming right away. But they didn't. It was radio silence - for two days straight, nothing at all. I couldn't believe it. I sat around in a daze in hooker makeup, regretting my decision and the money I had spent to change my airfare. What was I going to do now! I started freaking out. Anxious thoughts drove me crazy.

Until I realized I had forgotten to include my phone number in my ad. Within five minutes of correcting the problem, my phone beeped whenever someone texted me, Brooke coached me on how to respond. She explained how to give a sensual massage, techniques, and timing. And then it was time to put my training into action. When the first client showed up, I shook nervously. Brooke told me not to say too much while he was outside, but to usher him in the door discreetly. I opened the door, revealing my lingerie-clad body. The man looked at me like he had just won the lottery. He exclaimed something about how hot I was. Instantly, I calmed down. I directed him to undress completely and lay face down on the table. I stepped out of the room while he undressed. Brooke was waiting for me.

"He's cute!" I whispered.

"Did you get the money?" she asked.

I extracted a wad of twenties from my bra.

"Good! Now take your hair out of that ponytail and get that top off!"

I unsnapped my bra and returned to the room. Even though he had paid for half an hour, Brooke instructed me to just rub his back for about ten minutes, then rub lots of warm oil all over his inner thighs before asking him to roll over. She said it was okay to finish after about 20 minutes. The session went wonderfully. The man couldn't stop saying how much he loved my body. He wanted to touch me everywhere. Brooke had said not to let them touch me under my panties or to suck on me unless I wanted them to, and that I should ask for an extra donation for that.

After the session, I wiped the man down with a hot towel,

directing him to let himself out. I went to the kitchen to scrub like a surgeon. Brooke was waiting for me.

"Welllll?"

"Oh my God, that was so fun!" I blurted.

Brooke laughed. "I knew you'd love it! You've been so sexually repressed your whole life. It's time to let that pent up energy flow, girl!

Over the next month, I saw 5-8 clients per day. I was on a mission to make money. In my mind, you grabbed as much money as you could, as quickly as possible. I had a goal: become a big wave surfer. And nothing was going to stop me from getting there. You have to fight to get anywhere in life, right? Thirty days of making money lay in front of me. The more I earned, the more time I would have for surfing. My phone didn't leave my hands unless I was using my hands to massage. I was willing to do whatever it took to make money. If a guy wanted me to rub him with my feet, or wanted to meet me first at a nearby cafe, or wanted additional pictures, I would accommodate. I was scared to lose business by not catering to the customer's desires. But I quickly found out that these kinds of customers were way more work. One request often led to another and, before I knew it, I had wasted half an hour texting someone only for him to ask for "full service" (sex) and for me to turn him down. Brooke intervened.

"You are doing exactly what you did with your yoga business. You are giving away way too much and devaluing yourself."

"But I don't want to lose customers."

"Believe me, there is an endless supply of men with wads of cash in their pockets, all just dying to get a handful of that booty. Just wait for the good customers. Believe me, you will end up making more money if you just ignore the flakes."

It took me a while to get the hang of "ignoring the flakes." I felt bad every time I refused to send another photo and someone called me a bitch. I hated upsetting anyone. They would ask, *do you do this or that,* and I would agree, even though I didn't want to.

"You can't do that to yourself!" Brooke chastised me.

"But I need the money."

"Girl, get it through your head, there is PLENTY of money out there. When you run out, you can just make more. There is a never-ending supply. What's the rush? Why do you need it all now?"

"Because I have a goal!"

"And what's the rush for the goal? Can't you just enjoy yourself?"

The concept seemed strange to me. Just enjoy the process of making money, or surfing, or anything? I knew I should, but I didn't know how.

But Brooke explained that many of the callers were just taking advantage of me. They just wanted photos to jerk off to and they were never going to show up. Some of them were getting off just texting a hot girl and making up fantasies in their heads. She said they will always try to push me to do more, always. Saying no was the only way of setting the parameters, so that we both could have a good experience.
It took some getting used to. I was scared they wouldn't want to come see me if I told them no they could not do such-and-

such with me, but that turned out not to be the case. They were always excited and satisfied with what they got.

I'd be lying if I said I enjoyed every minute of it. I didn't. Some of the men drove me insane. They'd ask a million questions, trying to get me to do sex acts with them that I didn't do. They would bargain with me on price. They asked if my boobs were natural and what my measurements were. It made me feel like a commodity. They might as well have been asking what materials I was made of and about my battery life. Frequently, men made an appointment only to no-call-no-show. Brooke explained that if they were so picky they would only see a girl with certain measurements then I should be picky too and see less superficial men. Again, I worried about turning down work even if it did feel degrading. It took me a while to manage this but the more I did the more I found that my clients improved and I still had plenty of people calling.

One time, I opened the door to a very nervous looking man who instantly demanded that I show him my tits. He hadn't even stepped across the threshold. I explained that my top would come off during the massage, but I didn't like his aggression.

He barked, "If you won't show me your tits, how do I know you're not a cop! I'm not going to pay you unless you show me your tits!"

I felt about two inches tall. My gut felt like there was something rotting in it. I had just cut my surf session short, spent an hour shaving, doing my hair and makeup, and setting up the massage room. Now, this dickhead was threatening to leave if I didn't whip off my top for him. I started crying right there, my hand still on the doorknob, as he threatened to turn around and leave. I couldn't let all that money just walk out the door. Tears in my eyes, I tugged at my top and quickly flashed the guy.

I started setting boundaries, which was something new in my life. I declined all the special requests. I also set boundaries with my prices. I told myself I would never offer a discount. I was a human being, and humans don't go on clearance. I was afraid of losing clients, but I stuck to my guns. And I did lose some clients. But Brooke was right; there were plenty more.

The more I received questions about *would I do this* or *how big are those*, the more I added info to the FAQ's on my website. I also added a note about respect, showing up on time, and keeping your appointment. I even got bold enough to raise my prices, calling my massage "A high-end service for the discriminating gentleman." Little by little, my clientele rose to the standards I set. My website and prices weeded out the clients I really didn't want anyway.

These realizations were pivotal for me: That I was worth whatever I felt I was worth. That money was abundant. That men would pay a great deal to spend an hour being touched by me. A shift was taking place in me. A feeling of self-dignity was settling over me.

At first, I wasn't surfing much, always trying to be near my phone in case I got a call, afraid to miss an appointment. I told myself I had come to California to work, so just buckle down and do it. There was no time for enjoying my life now. That would come later. I was scheduling six appointments per day, finding no time for anything else, and running myself ragged. Slowly, I started declining clients, saying that I was booked for the day. By "booked" I meant that I had already seen enough clients and had made enough money for the day. I wanted to go surfing. I realized that most of the time, the guys would want to see me badly enough that they would make an appointment for a date in the near future. Soon, I was scheduling a week out. I was able to plan my day around my surf sessions and still make my goal income for the day.

That is when I began to really like my new work. The better my clientele became, the more time I made for myself, the better quality massages I was able to give. And as the quality of my service improved, I gained a steady clientele of repeat business and recommendations.

With each appointment, I grew to love my new, larger body even more. Men loved my soft belly and my round butt. They asked me to turn around and wiggle my ass. They said I was so sexy they couldn't stand it. They practically threw money at me to be touched. Ten years earlier, I believed I was too ugly and fat to be attractive. Nobody looked twice at me. I married a guy who told me that I wasn't attractive, but I would do. Less than two years earlier, I was desperately trying to lose weight to keep my next husband interested in me. Now I felt like Aphrodite, the queen of sensuality herself. And the only thing that had changed was my weight - the extra 30 pounds I had *gained*. That, and my confidence. It was now crystal clear to me: sexy was not about how I looked on the outside but what I believed I was worth. And at my hourly rate, I was starting to see just how much I was worth, indeed.

After a month of that work, my attitude greatly shifted about not only my body, but also money. *I am worthy, and there is always enough for me.* As soon as I embodied these truths, they were reflected to me in greater measure. I realized that there was plenty of money out there. I could have as much of it as I wanted. And I deserved it. Everyone does. The only thing that limits us from having the things we want in life is an attitude of unworthiness.

Still, I carried a lot of guilt about how I spent that month. I hated lying to people about what I was doing. But I couldn't risk telling anyone. The massage was just what I did in secret, and it wasn't legit. Perhaps a massive social media following and a status as one of the top female athletes in the world would do it for me. One by one, my struggles were vanishing. Yet the anxiety still lurked in the shadows.

The summer surf season was ending, but my big wave lust consumed me. I was starting to see some success in heavier waves. I desperately wanted to continue my training. The best place in the world for big wave surfing in the winter season is the North Shore of Oahu. I had been there once before, when I married Kurt. I placed a test ad for sensual massage on the Oahu websites. The next morning I woke up to 32 missed calls and texts from the Hawaii area code. My next move was clear.

I moved to Hawaii that winter and began surfing a couple of big wave spots. I got some really nice photos on some pretty big waves, enough to encourage me to keep going. My social media following jumped from 2k to 6k after a couple of particularly successful big wave sessions with photos. It was working, I was starting to live my dream! The money was good, the waves were good, my confidence was growing. I only had to work a few hours per day and I was still able to put large amounts of money away for whatever big surf trip would come next. I even started dating a retired pro surfer with a mansion on the beach. Sometimes strangers recognized me in public from Instagram. If I'm honest, this recognition felt even better than the waves I was surfing. With my free time, I started a blog about my surfing adventures and my struggles with food and body image. A few emails started coming in about how inspiring I was and my writing helped them

This should be where happily ever after comes in--at least for most people - money, romance, adventure, stability, recognition, influence. What could be better than making six figures, working part-time, dating a millionaire with major connections in the surf industry, and watching your own success and fame increase from doing what you love all the while helping and inspiring people?

I don't know what could be better. But there must be something because some large part of me still felt like I was letting down the entire human race. My lifelong anxiety wasn't placated. I wasn't doing enough with my life. I wasn't changing the world. Guilt filled me constantly about how I was making my money. I felt like my life was one big secret. How was I supposed to help people if I was lying to everyone about what I was? Plus, I knew that sensual massage was a time-limited career; I would age out after less than ten years. Then what would I do? I felt I should be saving and investing my money, not spending it on surf trips. I felt I should be earning more. Although I had grown, the question still haunted me. *Will there be enough?*

My body wasn't cooperating, either. Although I realized men didn't care nearly as much as I thought they did, living in Hawaii was hard on me. Everywhere I turned, some tiny little girl in a bikini was doing a photo shoot. I was afraid to eat anything out of the ordinary. Each week, I cooked seven chicken breasts and seven sweet potatoes. Every morning I made a salad, then the next three meals would be identical: ⅓ of a chicken breast, ⅓ of a sweet potato and salad. Over four months, I rarely varied my routine. But the cellulite would not be banished.

I didn't want any friends or family to come visit me. I was afraid they would find out what I was doing for money. I kept to myself around town because it was extremely hard to explain to anyone why I had so many clients all the time. I was constantly attached to my phone. I'd often have to leave friends abruptly to take a client. This made it quite difficult to maintain a social life. I was lonely and guilty. My mother called me one day to say she was concerned about how I was only living for myself. She said that "surfing isn't glorifying the Lord!" Even though I hated her for saying this, she was really only saying what I already believed about myself: that I was screwing everything up. I was supposed to be helping people, Instead, I was rubbing balls and splashing around in the ocean. I explained to her that my plan was to use the social media influence which I was growing to help empower women. But I'm not sure who I was trying to convince, her or myself.

Waves are seasonal. Some geographical locations pick up north swells and have waves in the northern hemisphere's winter months. Other locations work better in the summer with south swells. The North Shore of Oahu works in the winter. As the winter season came to an end, I thought ahead to where my next great adventure might take place. I was longing to get back to the freedom I tasted in Mexico. But this time I craved a new adventure. Every serious surfer eventually travels to Indonesia. I was ready to make my pilgrimage.

I was sharing lunch with my boyfriend when I broke the news that I had purchased a ticket to go to Indo. I told him I wanted more opportunities in big waves, which was part of the truth.

"Why do you want to ride big waves? You didn't start surfing as a kid. You are older now. Just leave that to the younger crew. Surfing should just be for fun. Why not just hang here with me? You could move in here. You could sit up in bed and check the waves at your favorite spot. You wouldn't even have to work anymore. Don't go to Indo. Stay with me." He grabbed my hand and looked me in the eyes. He had never been this straightforward with me before. I didn't know he felt that strongly for me.

But I knew what I wanted. And I knew, just like all the rest, he could not give me *happily ever after* either. I had to find that within myself. And unless I did, our relationship would never be what I knew some relationships hold the potential to be.

Chapter 30: Driven

When your source of happiness lies outside of yourself, it will always stay there, just out of reach, no matter where you go.

Indonesia was beautiful, of course, and the waves were incredible, of course. But I showed up with strep throat, which led to a weakened immune system. I was feeling run down and tired the moment I stepped off my second ten-hour flight. But I didn't let that stop me, even when it should have.

After saving money all winter in Hawaii,I had come to Bali on mission: to improve my surfing. The waves were more manageable than the big waves in Puerto or the heavy waves in Hawaii and the surf season was in full swing. So I had to surf, even if I wasn't feeling well. I found an incredible surf coach. Every session, I felt improvement. I needed to improve if I was going to ride big waves. This coaching was essential to my goal. And the waves were good.

Good waves can be so fickle. You can go months without good waves. It can be windy, the swell can be crossed up and bumpy, there could be no swell at all, the water could be dirty from the rain, the crowds could make it impossible to catch a wave, the swell could be too big for the location or too small or at the wrong angle, the tides could be wrong at the time of the day when the winds are right. There are dozens of factors that need to line up for good surfing. And so we wait, and we travel, and we rehearse on crappy conditions and we arrange our entire lives and sacrifice money and relationships and jobs and families in order to surf when the conditions *are* good. If we were to calculate how much money and time is spent on each good wave...well, we just don't do that. So I had to surf, no matter how I felt.

It started innocently enough, my slipping back into old food control patterns. I was traveling with a friend, so we coordinated meals together. She wasn't hungry in the morning before surfing, but I was. We would run out at dawn and surf four hours on empty stomachs. After a late post-surf breakfast, I was ready for a light lunch by mid-afternoon. But she didn't seem to be hungry yet. So, I distracted myself from the hunger by hitting the beach for some sprints or yoga, delaying lunch all the way until dinner. Once again, I would be truly hungry by the time dinner came around. And it felt so amazing. The food in Bali was incredible. The restaurants had amazing ambiance, and the presentation of the food was beautiful. Since I was truly hungry, I truly enjoyed my food. I ate slower and tasted it more than ever before.

After several days of this routine, my body realized it wasn't being properly fed. It threw a protest. Overtraining and underfueling had weakened my already weak immune system. I became quite ill, with a fever and vomiting. I had contracted a mosquito-borne virus similar to Dengue. While not as severe as Dengue, the symptoms of my virus persisted off and on with a fever recurring every few days for nearly four months. But I returned to my routine within merely four days, as soon as the vomiting stopped. The daily routine always included: a warm-up (100 squats and 100 crunches, a three to five-minute breath-hold), then surfing for three to four hours, then one hour of dry-land Crossfit style training and, lastly, sixty minutes of yoga. All on two meals a day. My abs once again rippled and my now much larger butt was still extra-large but no longer jiggly. It felt like victory.

Then my heart started to act funny.

It felt like my heart was being squeezed. I got lightheaded, and then it would be done. It would return at random times, maybe ten times in thirty minutes, and then not again for several hours. I noticed a lot of swelling in my legs. But nothing hurt. So I went surfing.

But my heart felt like it was pounding. My body felt weak and shaky. I cut my session short. And I felt guilty for doing so.

I got out of the water and felt hungry, truly hungry. But instead of going to get lunch, I decided to sit down and write for a while. I had surfed only one hour, and that wasn't enough to really earn a meal. *I can't risk getting fat. I need either to surf three hours or else not eat. I'm probably just feeling emotionally hungry.* It was confusing as I tried to battle against my body after having just learned so much about listening up.

The next day, the waves were good. I had a session scheduled with my coach. I had to surf. I just had to. My heart felt funny throughout the entire session, but I refused to tell my coach because I knew he would tell me to go in.

In 8th grade, my first basketball coach presented the end-of-year awards. He called my name to come up and receive the "Most Improved Player" award/insult. Before he shook my hand, we posed for a photo. He told everyone that, on my first day of practice, I threw the ball at the backboard so hard that it bounced to the other side of the court. It has always seemed to me that the right combination for success is brute force and sheer determination. Forcing the body to get the job done.

As politely as possible, my surf coach commented on my performance that day. "I don't know how else to say this, but your surfing looks like you are trying to lift heavyweights. You need to relax and not try so hard. Just flow with the waves." But flowing was not something in which I was well versed.

I began to notice that the more competitive the line up

became--the more people that paddled for the same wave--or the more I felt I was being watched, the harder I tried and the worse I performed on the wave. I was surfing with a girlfriend. I watched her surfing decline when she became frustrated with herself and forced herself to surf longer and harder without taking days off to rest. I saw how unhappy she was because she couldn't get her body to do what she wanted it to do. I saw her coming in from surfing frowning rather than smiling. I saw her beating herself up and, as a result, not having any fun in the water. It seemed ridiculous to me.

One afternoon, my chest started to feel as if it was being stabbed. Pain shot down my left arm. I hired a driver to take me two hours into town so I could see a doctor. A few hours later, hooked up to an EKG machine, I finally admitted how poorly I had been treating myself. I was still living out of fear: not enough time, not enough waves, and I was not enough. And then I saw it. I had exchanged one form of body control for another. I no longer vomited in order to have the best figure so everyone would see me and love me. But now I surfed and trained until exhaustion in order to get good photos on waves, so everyone would see me and love me.

I still didn't trust my body. I still wanted to be in control. I wanted to tell my body that it will surf for four hours and it will improve at surfing and it will be lean and muscular. And I'm right, I am. I can be lean and muscular and I can force my body to listen. I've done it before...and then I have cardiac distress. The body always gets the last word.

Upon their creation, God commanded humans to "fill the earth and subdue it," says the first chapter of the Bible. Live upon the earth with a sense of domination and exploitation, says the tradition I was raised in. Fear the earth, fear nature, tame it, and become powerful over it so it can't hurt you. The earth is a dangerous place, just waiting to destroy you should you let your guard down. And so is my body.

Heaven is the place you go when you die. You have just this one shot, this one very short life and then it is all over. Carpe Diem. Don't waste a moment. Fear time, for it is always ticking away. Accomplish now, push harder, be more. Train harder, surfer longer, be more influential, leave your mark on this earth. Don't waste a moment!

But surfing is about surrender. Control doesn't work in the ocean.

I have the power to control my body. Sure, I can force it to eat or not to eat. I can force it to move or not to move. I can restrain it from sex and food, I can force it to earn money. But at some point, my body wins. Nature always wins. There is an order to the universe. Fighting against the power of the ocean is a fool's errand, doomed to failure. I cannot control how long I am under water after a wipeout. I cannot control how fast I improve at surfing. I cannot control when the good waves come to me. I can train and practice, but there is so much more to surfing than the few factors I can control.

I have to let the wave do its thing, and then respond. The more I try to force maneuvers, the more I try to force my surfing prematurely, the worse I perform. The ocean is in control. The universe has a plan. It is not mine to control. I can fight all I want, but I will lose the battle. The ocean will always win.

Control. I don't have it. I hate that. Leaning into the discomfort of complete and total lack of control. I can't control how fast my surfing improves any more than I can control how the waves break. I can't control the weight at which my body is happiest. I can't control the speed at which recovery happens. I hate myself for mistreating myself. So I mistreat

myself for hating myself. Give it up.
after either. I had to find that within myself.

Chapter 31: Cookies

After my Indonesian visa expired I wanted nothing more than to return to Mexico. As Mexico always does, it settled me. I surfed and trained hard. I found more success, more photos, more big waves. There were lots more adventures in a camper van I picked up, and more flings with dark-skinned surfer boys. Everything was going according to plan...except for the anxiety, boredom, and loneliness of the long hot days when the wind turned onshore and there was nothing to do, stuck at home or confined to the bed in my van.

On the day before my birthday, I asked the universe for two birthday gifts: a barrel and good sex. Neither are hard to find in Puerto Escondido. As I exited a barreling wave, I saw him in the lineup. I knew him from last year and I knew exactly what was going to happen that night. Game on! It went so well in fact that I canceled an airline ticket I had purchased to visit a man in Spain. The next three months with my absolutely gorgeous, Afro-Mexicano Latin lover were nothing short of a dream. Every moment with him was like something out of a romance novel. It was so beautiful that it was heartbreaking. Oh, the sex! Three times a day, each time more intense than the time before. He was fiercely aggressive and loved to show me how much he wanted me. Not only did he have 8-pack abs and loved to dance, but he was also a phenomenal cook. He used the recipes his mother had taught him, preparing me beautiful, made-from-scratch, Mexican cuisine twice daily.

We saluted every morning with cookies from a glossy plastic sleeve. We ate a few cookies, sipped coffee, and headed out to surf. After surfing, he would prepare a massive breakfast of eggs, tortillas, and homemade salsa. We'd spend the hot afternoons napping and making sweet love. In the evenings, he'd cook again. I never wanted to snack because I so looked forward to his meals, each made with love. I wanted plenty of room to enjoy an abundant portion. Hunger felt like something to look forward to. After dinner, we'd go out dancing or stay in watching movies--with English subtitles when I was too tired to think in Spanish anymore.

Each day for three months, I would go to the market to buy a few cookies and a half kilo of warm tortillas. I never considered how much I was eating. I was in love. My weight didn't matter. I ate until I was full, and I looked forward to the next time I would be hungry. One time I mentioned that I felt I was a bit plumper. His response was so funny it immediately set me at ease.
"Calmate Natasha!" (Calm down Natasha!)

Something strange was happening. The feeling of hot restless energy in my sternum no longer felt like hunger. It felt like a sex drive. My new man was happy to satiate my hunger. Before long, my lover's diet of cookies, Mexican food, mind-blowing sex, and absolutely no stress dropped me to my lowest weight in several years.

One day, we had sex in a strange position that hurt my lower back. He asked if I wanted him to stop, but I enjoyed the pain (Of course I did). So I asked him to keep going. The next day, I couldn't sit or surf. The pain in my coccyx grew worse over the next few days. It was keeping me out of the gym and out of the water. I assumed it would heal in a few weeks. It would be nearly six months later when an x-ray showed the coccyx was broken. But shortly after the incident, I spent the afternoon skateboarding. When I got home, my entire back was aching worse than I had ever experienced. I put some ice on it and laid down. It wasn't the first time my back had gone out. It had happened at least two or three times over the last four years. I assumed, like the times before, it would resolve itself with rest over a matter of days. But the pain persisted. I was forced to modify my activity level further still.

After three months with my lover, it became clear we were cut from two different cloths. The cultural differences were too strong. I required creature comforts, while he was content to subsist. His approach to life was refreshing at first. He felt no one should worry about a place to lay his head or a meal; that as long as you just stayed present in the moment, all your needs would be met.

The truth is that he was right. But I wasn't accustomed to sleeping in hammocks and waiting on someone to pull up a fish to satisfy the rumbling in my stomach. My boyfriend didn't mind living like that in the least, which meant if I wanted a bed to sleep in and reliable meals I ended up paying for both our room and board.

It turned out that he, too, was an alcoholic. Why I always choose the alcoholics is still a mystery to me, but I do. Discovering his alcoholism was devastating but undeniable. He was stealing money from me and lying to me. I was being taken advantage of. I didn't want to believe such an amazing human could turn into such a monster by substance abuse, but I had seen it before and knew I had to face the facts. I wasn't going to do this to myself again. I told him it was me or the booze. And, like they always do, he said he would quit. Three days later, he was drunk again. I said it was his last chance, like I've said so many times before. I gave him about four last chances. Finally, he got drunk and stayed out until 4:00 am the night before a major surf competition for which I'd been helping him train for months. I packed my bags. The surf season in Mexico had come to an end anyway. At least this time it took me only a few weeks of hoping for the best before I faced the facts and cut ties. Heartbroken, I headed to Michigan to spend the holidays with my family.

I arrived back home in Michigan with perfect timing. My

mom was sick and needed significant help around the house for the holiday season. My back still throbbed, but I ignored it and pushed through. My mom needed my help. For the next six weeks, from Thanksgiving until the new year, I played Mom's role for the entire family. The cooking, cleaning, decorating, gift buying, wrapping, light hanging, errand running, caretaking of the farm, rental property and my elderly grandparents all fell on me. My mom had meticulously created a life devoid of free time for feeling the anxiety that lived just below the bustle. And with such a busy schedule I too found it easy to ignore the pain in my back and the anxiety in my heart. Some apples don't fall far from the tree.

One of my mom's first requests was for me to bake cookies. Not just any cookies; her gooey, chocolate chip, M&M, peanut butter, oatmeal cookies. Imagine all of the best kinds of cookies, all smashed into a single dough, and you have my mom's signature "monster" cookies. If these cookies are not heaven, then I don't know what is. I tucked an ice pack into the waistband of my pants to soothe my aching back and set to fulfilling my mom's request.

I love cookies. They are my favorite food. I have absolutely no defense against homemade cookies. As I mixed the dough, I pinched off a bite here and there. I put the unbaked portion of the dough into the fridge, to bake later. Over the next week, I went back for the raw dough at least once daily. The cookies became my daily breakfast, replacing the store-bought cookies with which I had greeted mornings in Mexico.

Staying at my parents is always a challenge to my willpower. There is a snack drawer. This evil drawer is filled with chocolate squares, granola bars, gourmet nuts, crackers, chips, popcorn, and all sorts of goodies I would never keep in my own home. On past visits, I would open the drawer as quietly as possible and when no one was looking. This time, I didn't really care who knew. I was constantly going in and out of drawers and cupboards, as I was now the matriarch of the kitchen. There was no one to stop me. And I was done policing myself anyway. If I wanted it, I could have it, guilt-free.

I decided to try an experiment I learned in a book called "Intuitive Eating". If I wanted to eat, then I would eat. When I read this book three years earlier it seemed absurd. But I was at last ready to listen to my body fully. Just like I had done in Mexico, I would eat when I was hungry and stop when I was full. I would eat anything that sounded good to me and not eat things that I didn't really care for. But without a breathtaking romance to calm my anxiety, replacing my Latin lover with my parents for roommates left me constantly hungry.

When Aunt Denise dropped off a plate of her signature Christmas cookies, I dug in. When Dad busted out the ice cream to watch his evening TV shows, I grabbed a bowl. When I picked up the gifts from my mom's students, I helped myself to the fudge. When I attended church with my parents, I laid into the doughnuts that were offered with the coffee. This went on for 6 weeks straight. For the first time in my life, I allowed myself unlimited sweets. I enjoyed every bite. At times I felt guilty, but I constantly reminded myself that this was my process. Six weeks later, when I stepped on the scale to weigh the bag I was taking with me to Hawaii, I had gained 15 pounds. Seeing the number was difficult, especially after feeling so proud of myself for losing so much weight in Mexico.

Self-loathing came on strong. But I made the mature decision to sit with it. I knew I had honored my body and my desire. I knew my body didn't feel entirely healthy, but I also knew the only way through this was right into the thick of it. Desire is good and can be trusted, I reminded myself. My desire was for cookies. I needed to become the cookie monster!

I left my parents in Michigan and arrived in Hawaii after the new year, enthused to have my own space back, and still craving cookies.

I decided if cookies were what I wanted, then I would have cookies. The heart is the roadmap to understanding and love. Unhealthy-seeming desires were healthy for me, at that moment. My heart wanted cookies. I went to the store with my mom's recipe in hand and purchased all the ingredients for the best cookies in the world. I went home and made a triple batch. I ate them for three meals per day, for three days until they were gone. I went back to the store and bought more ingredients. The next triple batched lasted a week.

The third triple batch lasted two weeks, until I had to discard what was left because they had a funny smell. I didn't make the cookies again for months. They simply didn't sound good. I could not believe it. All those eating disorder books had been right, all along. If I simply ate what I wanted, even if it seemed "unhealthy" or "excessive", eventually my body would even itself out. Unfortunately, with cookie cravings gone and my aching back precluding exercise, l was again filled with anxiety. But, for the first time, the anxiety felt a lot more like anxiety and a lot less like cookie cravings. I considered this to be a step in the right direction.

I assumed the 15 pounds would come off when it was ready. Some days it bothered me, other days it didn't. I was back to working, doing massage, and no one seemed to mind the extra plump ass. At least I could always count on my clients to validate me. And returning to surfing at the height of big wave season on Oahu meant that plenty of new men approached me from all sides. I let myself have as many sex partners as cookies if that was what I wanted.

But letting myself off the hook to not surf for a time while my back healed was still beyond my maturity level. Pain in my back had persisted for over three months now. Basic motions like sitting twisting and bending were always bothersome. I was forced to cut my surf sessions short. I wasn't able to run or lift weights. I even had to refrain from many traditional yoga poses. I tried resting the best I could but found it very anxiety-producing to stay still for too long. I knew I probably should take some time off from surfing but just the thought of it was heartbreaking. Plus the extra cookie weight was making it difficult to look in the mirror. I wanted it gone, but the weight wasn't going to fall off of me while I laid on my ass. So I pushed through the pain.

One day, a guy I had known a few years ago back in San Diego spotted me on the beach. I had been feeling particularly horrible about my weight that day. We had never really talked much except for saying hello in the water of the parking lot. Out of nowhere, he called out to me as I passed by.
"Hey Nat, I just wanted to tell you... well...your body is looking amazing right now!"
He didn't even seem to be hitting on me. It was weird. It was like he had just seen a handsome dog or an amazing sunset and was simply remarking on its beauty.
"Thanks, I needed to hear that today," I told him. As I walked away, I had no idea how much the comment would turn my life upside down forever.

Chapter 32: Sex

All I knew was that as much as I no longer felt guilty for eating cookies, neither did I feel guilty for having casual sex, and that I very much enjoyed it. It wasn't the actual orgasmic experience of sex that I craved. For if it had been, I easily could have satisfied that craving by myself. What I really enjoyed was being desired. That was the best anti-anxiety medication (apart from food and movement) I had found. The approval of men meant something. The ruling class desired me. My beauty was enough to validate me. It also meant security. If I was valuable enough for men to want me, then I had options for my future. I could be with a rich guy. Or I could continue being a high-end sensual massage therapist charging far more than the market rate, exclusively choosing only the clients I really wanted to work with, even charging them extra for "extra" if I was horney, the guy was hot and nice enough, and it sounded fun to me. There would be nothing more to worry about; happily, ever after seemed to be held in my sexual power.

I had learned one valuable lesson in my recovery: if my heart wanted to do it, then it would ultimately lead to goodness, even if it seemed an unlikely path. Even if I caused myself great hurt in the process. If I wanted something, that desire wasn't going away until I acted on it. I might as well get it out of my system. Denying desire is a recipe for powerlessness. And I had desires.

That winter in Hawaii, I aimed to get enough photos and videos of me surfing big waves to earn an invitation to the XXL Big Wave Tournament. The tournament took place in Puerto Escondido the following summer. My back pain was limiting the number of hours I could spend surfing. Not having to get up in the morning to spend hours training meant I was looking for something else to fill my time, and hold back my anxiety. Drinking was an easy option. One night I was at a house party. Pro surfers and their entourages swarmed the place. As in a surfing line up, the ratio of guys to girls at the party was stacked heavily in my favor. I reveled in the attention, dancing sexily in the middle of the room. But I let no one touch me, keeping my options open. After a couple of hours of soaking up as much attention as I could, something struck me: I could have pretty much anything I wanted. That excited me. I cultivated the thought. I decided I was ready to get laid. I checked in with myself. Am I going to regret this? FUCK NO! I looked around the room. There were so many options. My eyes darted back and forth. I couldn't decide between two very young, dark-skinned, heavily muscled surfer boys. Both had deep brown eyes, rippling shoulders, and abs. I couldn't make up my mind. I honestly resorted to *eenie meenie minie moe*. The 21-year-old from Tahiti won the game.

The Tahitian broke off from the group to grab another drink. I approached him. I kept it short and sweet. "I'm going home now. Come over in 10 minutes...if you want." I lived just a few houses up the street.

Two minutes after I got home, the door opened. There he stood. His clothes came off and mine followed. No words were required. Unfortunately, being 21, within four minutes he was sprawled across the bed, breathless and glassy-eyed. I was cracking up.
"You gotta be kidding me! You got another round in you, right?" I exclaimed through my laughter.

"Yeah, but I got an idea. What do you think about Kalani?" Kalani had been the other option in my game of *eenie meenie minie moe*.

"He's hot!"

"Want to have a threesome?" he asked.

"Go get him!" I shot back.

Fifteen minutes later, my legs spread wide as two 21-year-old professional athletes ravished my naked body.

The next morning, I woke up alone. The memory of the night before was fresh in my head. I groped around under my pillow for my vibrator. Suddenly, the door to my studio apartment was flung open. There stood the Tahitian.

"Can I come in?"

I smiled and pulled back the covers, revealing my still naked body.

"Get in here, I was just thinking about you!" I grinned from ear to ear. *I deserve all of this and more.* I returned to bliss.

Two days later, early in the morning hours, another pro surfer from the party the other night showed up at my door. He wasted no time in telling me what he wanted. Word must have gotten out about my sexual availability. But I wasn't in the mood nor attracted to him. He begged and wouldn't leave. I eventually gave in just for the sake of being nice. I felt icky inside when it was over. I didn't even have an orgasm. I recommitted myself to my own happiness first, even if it meant bruising a man's ego. A few days later he returned, hungry for more. But this time I knew what I did and did not want and I stuck to it. I had to physically turn his shoulders around and send him on his way. I felt incredibly rude.

Something inside of me was unsettled about the kind of sex I was having. I had come to believe that desire was the path to unleashing the greatest power. And I desired sex. So I indulged in it. But it was like feeding stray cats. They just kept showing up for more. One night, a man I had previously slept with entered my unlocked apartment while I was sleeping in bed with another man. The first man laughed and turned around. Another late night, two guys banged on my door. They wanted another threesome. I was getting sick of all the strays looking for another handout. But I hated saying no. I didn't want to hurt their self-esteem. I didn't want to make them mad. And, looking back, I can see that I didn't want to lose my power over them.

The Brazillian asked if I wanted to go surfing with him. It was big and kinda bombing the day we met up. We sat on the beach looking at the surf. He kept trying to grope me on the public beach. I was annoyed. I'd only just met him (at church, actually) and this was our first time hanging out together. He was copping a feel within 15 minutes. I knew how much I charged men to feel me up, and this man was getting something for nothing.

We surfed for a couple of hours. He showed me how to ride the inside barrel section while he sat on the outside and took some 20-foot drops.

"I think you are a good enough surfer to date me," he said after his session.

Are you kidding me? I wanted to smack the guy! But instead, I faked a giggle.

I was ready to go home but he wanted to get lunch. We grabbed some take out. I paid. Then, we stopped by his house for him to grab something before returning to the beach to eat. He asked me to come inside with him. I knew that put me in a vulnerable situation. I didn't trust his aggression. I said I'd wait in the car.

"Just come in with me. What's the big deal?"

Apparently, no didn't really mean no with this guy. I gave in. I wanted to be *nice*.

He rented a tiny room and there was no place to sit, so I stood. He told me to sit on the bed. I said I was good. He pulled gently on my arm. I yielded. He began kissing me. I clearly stated, "I don't want to fuck right now." He said he just wanted to cuddle. I didn't want to cuddle, but I let him pull on my body until that was what we were doing.

Before I knew it, his hand was in my pants and my animal urges kicked in. I stopped trying to fight him and let myself enjoy it. His style was brutal. Surfers fuck like they surf, and he was an animal in the water. He called me a whore. I felt like one, and I liked it.

"Do you wanna be my slut? Do you want me to bring my friends and let them all fuck you?"

I said I did, and I meant it. Being brutalized in that moment, I was his, I belonged to him. My dirty evil body deserved to be treated like the whore it was. YES, everyone, come fuck the shit out of this stupid body that I've always hated anyway. At least I can give it to you for your entertainment. Take me. I'm worthless anyway. Your desire for me gives me value. You are the man, and am just the worthless woman. Use me!

He enjoyed me long after my enjoyment ended, twice.

After we were done, my body felt like it had been beaten up, because it had been. We went to the beach for lunch, even though what I really wanted was to go home and be away from him. We fell asleep on the beach even though I wanted to go home and be productive with my afternoon. I woke up to the feeling of his weight over me. I protested, not here, not now, someone might see. He promised he'd be quick.

He had a party to go to that afternoon and he wanted me to come with him. I didn't want to go, but I couldn't find my no. I resigned myself to the fact that this would be my entire day, even though I had other things I wanted to do. We went to the store to buy some snacks and beers for the party. I paid again.

Dropping me off after that evening, he invited himself into my house. I said I just wanted to go to bed. He said he just wanted to see my place. Three rounds of slapping, choking, and spitting later, he left and I passed out.

One month earlier, while visiting my parents, I was sitting in the church I grew up attending. Five beautiful sisters sat in the row in front of me. Aged from 13 to 21, they all looked alike: modestly dressed with decorative clips in their long, blond, wavy hair. I watched them as the pastor droned on and on about being nice when people are mean to you. I wondered if these girls would grow up to be kind, like the pastor said Jesus asked us to be, even when people treated us really badly. Jesus let his body be spit on and let himself be brutalized. But he was still kind and never resisted.

Sitting on my outdoor couch, the day after my explosion of nonconsensual sex, I thought of those girls. Inside, the Brazilian stretched out on my bed. He said he wanted to come over, just to talk. I gave in and agreed, just to talk. When he started grabbing me, I momentarily stopped him with a firm no. But he came back at me.

"I'm serious. I don't want to fuck and I don't believe you when you say you just want to kiss, and I don't want you to touch me!" I didn't say it nicely. And I was distinctly unkind as I shoved his body off of mine.

"Okay, I won't touch you." He extended his index finger toward me, mimicking a poke, mocking me.

"You can stay and hang out if you want," my nice Christian girl said, "But I have work to do." The wiser part of me picked up my computer and went outside to work on the porch. He promptly used my bed for a two-hour nap, then gathered his things and left, promising to call me tomorrow. My Christian girl smiled and let him kiss me goodbye.

I kept him in my back pocket for months. I actually felt that I'd like to have sex with him again. The brutality of the encounter reminded me of the way my parents loved me and how they said God loved me. Love meant following the rules. Love was control. Love was punishment. Love was pain. So, of course, sex would embody these ideas. Some primal part of me loved being taken advantage of. It seemed to validate all the deeply conditioned beliefs about the roles of men and women that still haunted my subconscious. Plus, having that kind of sex felt like a big "Fuck you" to all the authorities who had told me sex was wrong. *I'll show you the wrong sex!*

Each time we fucked, he used words like, "Do you like being raped by me?" And my honest answer was yes. I told him to hit me harder. My neck was bruised the next day from his choking. He called me a slut and a whore and it made me go crazy. Yes, I am, yes I am, yes I am!

Why was something so brutal so pleasurable for me? How did I go from not wanting it to wanting more of it? Sex is wrong. Loving sex feels like an oxymoron. When you still can't quite wrap your head around what healthy sex really is, dirty nasty fucking makes a whole lot more sense than making love.

Each time I saw him, I felt awful afterward. But I kept wanting more. Is it like eating cookies, I wondered? If I give myself unconditional permission to eat as many as I want, will I eventually stop wanting to eat them? If I enjoy sex with as many partners as I want, fulfilling all my dirtiest fantasies, will I eventually crave a more stable and loving sex life?

He invited himself over. But I didn't want him there. I said he could come in for just a minute. I was certain I did not want to have sex with him that night. He shoved me down on the bed. I pushed him off with a nervous giggle and a weak throated "nooo".

"Don't worry, I just want to kiss you a little. I won't do anything you don't want." He promised this as he shifted his weight on top of me.

I tried squirming away as he reached his hand up my shirt. He got the point and instead gripped my thighs.

"No," I stated weakly, "I don't want to. My back hurts today." The truth was my back was hurting worse than ever, and I didn't feel up for sex at all. That afternoon I had been surfing in Waimea Bay when a triple overhead wave had exploded in my back sending me flying forward in the shape of a scorpion. I couldn't sit, stand or move without severe pain. I had an ice pack on my back as I rested in my bed. I had been crying most of the day from the pain and the sneaking suspicion that something was seriously wrong with my spine.

"I'll be gentle," he assured me, softly rubbing a finger over my cotton shorts. I moaned a little as blood started flowing down there. He took it as a green light.

Two minutes later, it wasn't gentle and I wanted out.

"You are hurting me," I stated it clearly.

But he kept at it, now removing my shorts as I winced and groaned from the pain.

"I don't want to do this right now," I repeated myself.

"I'll give you a massage afterward," he said as he unzipped his pants and entered me. I cried out in pain.

"But I'm almost there!" he countered.

"I don't want to keep doing this. It hurts. I am in pain." I emphasize my point in no uncertain terms. I tried to squirm away from beneath him but the movements hurt worse than just lying still.

"Just five more minutes." He rammed his hips into me even harder.

"I want to stop!" I nearly shouted and pushed against him.

He sat up for a minute, smiled, and then went back to his business. I let my body go limp, gritted my teeth, and looked away.

He finished the job and walked to the bathroom, a big smile on his face. "Wow. baby. You turn me on so much."

When he said this, the strangest thing happened inside me. I knew how angry I had the right to be, in fact, needed to be. At 34 years old, this was far from the first time I had failed to stand up for myself. I knew that, if I didn't get angry at that moment, I would allow something similar to happen again and again. A sweet-as-apple-pie smile was pasted onto my face. But I forced my jaw to soften, erasing the facade.

"That wasn't cool." I blurted out. *Come on Natasha, you can do better than that!*

"What do you mean? I didn't do anything." He looked genuinely confused.

Come on, get mad. It's down there, feel it. Intellectually, I reminded myself that I had just been violated--I needed to activate anger. I reached into a deeper place than I normally can access. I noticed something hot and turbid down there.

"The very fact that you don't think you did anything wrong when you didn't stop after I asked you to is what makes me angry!" I forced myself to speak these words loudly. It felt completely unnatural to speak in such a harsh tone of voice.

"Baby…" He tried to get back in bed with me.

"Don't touch me!" I hissed and backed away quickly. "I'm pissed at you. You need to leave. Now!" I felt like I was reading theater lines. I knew I needed to say them. I knew they needed to be said the way I was saying them, but the anger behind them just wasn't there. I couldn't reach deep enough to experience it.

I instantly felt bad for my words, but reminded myself that they were warranted.

He sat on the couch across the room and apologized…insincerely. The longer he spoke, the more I tried to feel the anger, but I couldn't reach it. I wanted to scream at him, "You just fucking raped me, you filthy motherfucker! Get the hell out of my home before I call the police!" I dug as deep as I could to find the same anger that had animated my tongue moments before, but it slipped just as quickly through my fingers. The nice Natasha had already resumed command. I politely listened for the next 15 minutes as he droned on about a religious topic he learned while in seminary school. Finally, as sweetly as possible, I told him I was really tired and I wanted him to leave so I could sleep.

"I'm just going to grab some water, is that cool?" He walked toward the kitchen, the opposite direction of the door.

"Go ahead." I laid back on my bed. I let my body go limp. A tear traced its way down my cheek.

It has always been about validation. I changed my physical body to gain attention from men. Subconsciously, I knew this. Weight loss had always been about gaining validation from men.

Looking for validation on the outside renders you powerless. If validation is found in an Instagram following, from winning beauty competitions, from men throwing themselves at me, then my power is in the hands of my followers, my judges, and those men. Something had shifted. I had grown too strong for this path.

Now I see that sex is the mingling of souls, I told my journal. *Choose wisely, sweet girl, who you let in... I'm over the sex, the parties, the attention. I don't want to set boundaries. I don't want to say no. I just want to be with someone who respects me enough that boundaries are not necessary. I am more than a body. I'm so sick of all this. They are just using me. And I guess I'm using them...I'm ready for a real partner. I'm ready to be with just one man who loves me, not ten men who love my body. I don't ever want to put myself in a position where I have to tell a guy no again.*

Finally, I had sown my wild oats. After 34 years, at last, I had granted myself permission to do what I wanted. And I did it, and it was great. And I no longer wanted to do that. I was satiated.

Now that junk food and meaningless sex had lost their ability to get me high, what was left to distract myself from my anxiety, from the debilitating fear that I would never be enough? Just one thing: Surfing big waves.

Chapter 33: Devastating Diagnosis

Waimea Bay and Sunset Beach became my obsessions. I surfed them both any chance I got. Going for a surf at these locations isn't your casual, every day, I just feel like getting wet, kind of surf. You have to study the forecast, when the swell will be building, what the tide is doing and what wind conditions will be. You don't want to be looking for medium waves on a rising swell with a dropping tide as you are sure to get caught by a bigger set forming out the back. You don't want to be sitting deepest when the wind switches to onshore, the current starts dragging you out to sea and there are no rideable waves to bring you in. Surfing at the edge of my comfort zone took the best of my mind and body. And it was addictive.

There is a feeling I get in my chest when I see the swell forecasted to be big. It is hot and restless. My heart pounds; I might call a friend to verify that winds and conditions will indeed be favorable. I don't sleep well the night before the swell. When I wake in the morning my bowels move faster than usual. My appetite is non-existent as I toss some small snacks in my bag and load my car. Wetsuit, impact suit, rashguard, big wave leash, wax, fins, fin key, 10'0" Dick Brewer. The feeling in my chest has slowly been growing but as I pull up to the beach It seems to explode as I watch the first set break in deep water. I sit to watch a few sets, determining how conditions look, what the current might be like, where I want to position myself, and if I truly want to go out at all. I control my breath. I watch. My thoughts are almost silent. I am looking and feeling, looking, and feeling. As the first surfers come in, I exit my car and begin to ready my surf tools. I ask them about their waves, about the current, about the wind. They seem 100 times more chill than I am pretending to be. My heart is racing. Anxiety is at an all-time high.

I'm an addict. If I'm not about to throw myself into a life and death situation, my mind will find another way to manufacture the same anxious feeling in my chest. Big waves are the interruption to the constant stream of thoughts reminding me I need to be doing more with my life. These thoughts give me the same jittery feeling that the waves produce. But when I'm staring into the face of death waves, the thoughts go on mute. It just feels right.

That day was a Waimea day. I drove to the beach alone. I was delighted to see a few familiar faces in the parking lot. These guys said the waves were perfect for me. My heart pounded. My back ached. Somewhere within me, I knew the dangers were increased due to my back pain which had now been quite strong for over three months. But the addiction won. As I entered the water my mind went blank. Inhale. Right arm. Exhale. Left arm.

At Waimea, because the wave is mostly just a drop-down terrifying face without much shoulder to ride, it is common for two or more surfers to share the same wave. The first wave I chose, I shared with four other surfers, I was the second from the last, meaning closer to the shoulder than the peak. This made the wave less steep, easier to catch, easier to ride. My confidence increased. The second wave I was a bit deeper, only one other person was closer to the peak than me. I saw the photographer in the water and made sure to get his contact info. That wave felt like heaven. I waited a long time for my third wave. After maybe forty minutes of waiting for the perfect wave, I was growing restless. Just then I saw the horizon starting to get dark. A set was coming. I had worked myself closer and closer to the peak. It was my turn. One of the guys sitting too far out to catch this wave looked back at me and nodded. That nod commenced the beginning of what would turn out to be the last big wave I have ridden. It might be the last I will ever ride.

I was the one on the peak this time. The woman who shared the wave with me surfed in front of me. She was closer than I felt comfortable with. In a split second my programming took over. *She can have the best part of the wave, I'll just straighten out. Yes, that will mean getting mowed over by the wave but I'll be fine. Don't worry about me, I just don't want to screw it up for someone else.* I never consciously thought of any of that, there wasn't time. There were just 34 years of conditioned response.

The MRI results were bad, much worse than I had anticipated. After the Waimea incident, I assumed the pain eventually would just go away. It had been almost six weeks since the lip of that extra-large wave exploded in my back. I felt something pop at that moment, and the pain that I had been experiencing for the previous three months multiplied and shot through my lumbar spine. After taking weeks to rest and complete physical therapy with no improvement, the doctor ordered the scan.

They wouldn't tell me over the phone. In the office, the doctor wouldn't even discuss with me the extent of the damage. She said she wasn't sure how I was even walking right now. She referred me straight to the spine surgeon. I held it together at the doctor's office but, as soon as I got in the car, I began beating the steering wheel and screaming at no one. I felt everything I had spent the last year and a half working toward slipping through my hands. My plan, my dream, was being wrenched from my grip.

I blew every disk in my lumbar spine.

I lost it right there in front of the World Surf League's Doctor when he said it would be a year before I'd surf again, and that I should forget ever surfing 30-foot waves.

I wandered around feeling lost for two days. Waves of nausea gripped my body and tears poured.

No no no! Don't take this dream from me!

This is all I have. I gave up everything, everything! I own nothing. I'm literally alone on a beach with no family or friends nearby, crying my eyes out with pain shooting through my body, hiding my tears under a hoodie from all the happy tourists walking by.

I push limits. I always have. I guess I found mine. Most people never do.
I was willing to do whatever it took. I put in more hours, I studied longer, I trained harder. I had to be vigilant. No moment went wasted.

I've never once done a single thing half-assed, in my entire life. And many times my best wasn't good enough, so I learned to do better. They told me I could do anything I wanted if I just worked hard enough. "I can do all things through Christ who strengthens me," the Bible said and my mom promised me. "You can do anything you set your mind to."

There was no risk I wasn't willing to take, no fear I wasn't willing to face. I am a master of self- discipline, mind over matter, and willpower. But it doesn't work that way. They were all wrong. Nature cannot be bullied. And, suddenly, I found myself sitting on the beach, watching the vastus lateralis muscle in my thigh spasm with excruciating pain. The reality is that I did it to myself.

The doctors shot some radiation through my body so they could look inside. They told me what I already knew: everything needs to change. My entire lumbar spine was severely damaged. There was tearing, bulging, herniation, nerve damage, and bone damage. This didn't happen overnight. Years and years of escaping my anxious thoughts by ignoring what I truly wanted and instead pushing my body to perform had finally caused debilitating damage. A combination of one big fall and one small one executed the finishing touches.

We caught it soon enough. I would not forever be disabled. But I had to change everything about the way I lived. I had to change who my ego said I should be. After several months of rest, the doctor said I would need several more months, even years, of physical therapy to change movement patterns I had developed over a lifetime. *But who will help me change the thought patterns?*

I told my parents I was thinking about going back to school to become a doctor. If surfing wasn't an option anymore, then I needed to find something else to give me a sense of purpose. My parents were thrilled. To be honest, the idea broke my heart. I looked at the surfers out on the water and thought about myself in a lab coat under a fluorescent light. My heart shattered into a million little pieces.

The crazy thing is, I didn't want to escape my emotion. I could have consoled myself. But I wanted to feel it. I even stopped eating very much. I wanted to be overtaken by emotion, and food would have numbed it. Sex sounded petty. I needed the reality of that moment and nothing else. I have always sought experiences at the fringe of human capacity. And no I was having one. I dared not shy away.

For days I lay around in pain and stunned silence. What are you, Natasha? What do you really have? Why are you here? What is the point?

All of life had conspired to get me to this place, and I had been running from it. I had turned to achievements, to food, to sex. You can only run from your destiny for so long. Life always finds a way. Unfortunately, I had chosen the path of resistance, and now I would have to walk through the pain that such a path brings. But I knew this experience was a compass to guide me to my deepest fulfillment, whatever that may be. One thing looked certain, it wasn't big wave surfing just as it hadn't been owning a yoga studio or being thin or having the right husband. Everything that had been taken from me was taken for a reason. The question became, would I be open to the path this pain asked me to walk next? Or would I fabricate another resistance plan?

Chapter 34: Awakening

"It is through gratitude for the present moment that the spiritual dimension of life opens up."
-Eckhart Tolle

I had a lot of time on my hands, unable to exercise, surf, or even work. Time slowed. Each moment deepened. If before big wave surfing had been my obsession I now diverted the newly freed up energy into mental recovery. I became obsessed with understanding what lesson I was meant to learn. But the only way I knew to do this was to lay still and listen. And it was working. Subtle shifts in the way I moved within my day startled me. I felt I was being reborn as a whole new person. And birth hurts.

I was in immense pain. I could see the pain was twofold, the physical pain from the injury and the mental pain from the story I had attached to it. I could choose to give up the story, even if I could not control my body. I could sit with it, explore it, write about it, dive in it, and hopefully learn something from it. But one thing was certain, I would learn nothing if I kept trying to talk over it, ignore it and cover it.

It took six days of mourning after receiving my MRI results before I began to pull myself toward the light. Historically, I had learned that the greater the hurt, the greater the joy on the flip side. I knew that each time when something I thought I could not live without had been taken away from me, I received something more fulfilling in return. Now my athleticism was ripped from my hands. My body, the thing I treasured (and hated) most, was gone. What gift could be waiting on the other side of this injury to replace my body? And I knew exactly what I had to do to get through this pain of loss. I had to make friends with it.

There would be no lasting happiness in the future. The past

had taught me this. I had to learn to fall in love with the present moment. No more numbing, no more running toward future results. No more using activity or exercise or food or sex or achievements to check out of the moment. But, of course, I was still naive about exactly how much pain this challenge would require. I oscillated by the hour between excitement over a brighter future and anger toward a seemingly unjust world. How could a career-ending injury be for my greatest good? I didn't know, but somehow my deepest being knew that it was.

Once again the ocean was the only force big enough to hold my pain. Although the one block walk to the water was often excruciating, I went to her daily, sometimes sitting beside her, sometimes entering her, but always spending the time with her that I would have if I had been surfing. Something primal within me was connecting through the water to a source greater than myself. I was floating in the ocean one afternoon, letting the salt water once again provide healing from the crushing force of gravity on my spine. I dove deep. From 10 feet below the surface of the water, I watched a wave crash over me. Frothy bubbles fizzed above me. Turquoise and faint purple glinted off the perfect impermanent spheres. Salt burned my eyes, my lungs asked to breathe. But neither the salt nor the urging of my lungs was enough to break me free of the spell of those tiny, fizzling orbs. *Is this what awake feels like*? I'd never before seen a wave break from that far below. I'd never appreciated how beautiful they are. I had always tried just to get on top of them and make them do something for me.

Clarity began to flood my life. It's sad that it takes a tragedy to appreciate what we have left. Riding big waves, getting photos, gaining a following, looking sexy in a bikini, having endless attention from men, what my mother thought of me...what had any of it gotten me? If I got in the ocean, that was enough. If I enjoyed each bite, that was enough. If I beheld the beautiful in the ordinary, that was enough. Could I watch waves break with as much enthusiasm as I used to ride them? Taking in their beauty became a brand new joy. Sex with people I didn't love no longer appealed to me. I began craving that one person with whom I could practice true, unconditional love, whoever he or she may be. As my life came to a screeching halt I noticed small moments of deep satisfaction in my everyday tasks, such as eating.

One day after finishing a meal, I leaned back in my chair and grabbed my chest. *That was intense!* Like collapsing on a lover, completely spent and satisfied. I released a huge sigh. For thirty minutes I had been entranced by a sensory overload. The sound of the sizzling onion and garlic, the smell of browned butter, the flakey texture of fish, the crunch-crunch of corn chips, the deep red of salsa, the zing of lime. All of my senses were at once sources of powerful pleasure. I ate quicker and quicker. Soon, the knife had been set aside and I cut everything with a fork to save time. I poured from the container of oil rather than drizzling. My crunching grew louder inside my head. The bites were faster and faster with less and less chewing between swallows. Until, boom! I swallowed the last bite. And then it all stopped. My plate was empty; the last bite had just been swallowed. No more sizzling, no more crunching. In the next split second, I stood and turned toward the stove for a second round of sensory explosion. But within that split second, there was the briefest moment of pause. Awareness leaped into the opportunity of that minute sensory pause.

It was the film flapping off the reel right at the climax of the movie. The screen fell instantly black and the room became silent. No more sizzling, no more crunching.

Whoa! Snapped from a trance, I stood in the kitchen sucking deep breaths and staring at the leftovers. A cold glass of consciousness splashed my face. I rose above my senses to notice my own reaction to the pleasure. I noticed how quickly I had just been eating, and how loudly the crunching still rang in my ears. I drew a single chip from the bag. I examined its rich blue color. I noted the texture of salt grains rubbing off onto my fingers. I held the chip to my nose and took in its scent. Then, I put the chip in my mouth and bit down. CRRRRUNCH. I bit down only once. I emitted an involuntary sigh of all-consuming satisfaction. CRUNCH CRUNCH CRUNCH! I chewed three times more. I giggled at the sound-- so fun! I began chewing so vigorously that, when I swallowed, my entire body moaned in pleasure.

I felt my hand reaching for another. I watched as my fingers grasped it. I rushed to get the chip into my mouth. I noticed how much I didn't notice the crunch this time as I hurried to get to the third chip, which was already in my hand. The chip was already on its way to my mouth before I'd even had a chance to finish enjoying what I was currently chewing. I stopped.

How much pleasure can I extract from each calorie? What If I'm not looking for nourishment right now, but pleasure? It was a moment of victory in the home stretch of half a lifetime's battle with food. *Could the pleasure I find in food be found elsewhere?*

I thought of many friends who completed 40-day fasts for religious reasons, and how they were just fine, physically. They didn't actually need to eat to survive. And in that moment, having just completed my third reasonably sized meal of the day, neither did I need to eat more food. So why did I still feel hungry? I was hungry for pleasure.

I thought of the chemistry I had with my Afro-Mexican lover. We spent every last minute wrapped up in each other's arms. For several days, we hardly ate a thing because we didn't want to. In love, we existed outside our humanity, the needs of the body masked by fulfilling the needs of the soul. We were so content to be naked in bed with each other that we couldn't be bothered with silly human things like eating. We were already gorging ourselves on pleasure.

I stood there in my kitchen, frozen halfway between my empty plate and the waiting leftovers, completely enraptured in a flash of consciousness. I became aware of the pleasure that had just passed and my desire for more. I simply held that desire for a moment, entirely curious about its sensation in my body.

As soon as it was over, a second helping would make me feel overly full. Then I would be standing in this same spot, wanting a third helping, grasping for more pleasure. I would feel guilty and "fat" (whatever that means), and still wanting more. The pleasure would not last, but could I find equally as much pleasure in some other way, in the next moment of my day?

Moving on to wash the dishes was the best answer. I enjoyed the warm water and soap sliding over my hands. I noticed the clinking of the dishes in the sink and the chirping of crickets outside. I wondered if one day I could find washing the dishes as satisfying as eating the meal.

And then I remembered those fucking eating disorder books I had read so long ago. They said that, when you feel a binge coming on, you should go for a walk or take a hot bath — *the fucking bubble bath*. I chuckled. *Oh my god, that's it*. It dawned on me, they were right all along! But I wasn't ready for them yet. First, I simply needed to learn that the universe was good, there was plenty of food and money, and my body and desires could be trusted. I learned this by eating...a lot. And by doing things I wanted to do rather than things I felt I *should* do. Specifically, by selling my yoga studio, traveling in Mexico, having sex, and making money doing sensual massage. Yes, I now faced some consequences, but this was my process. At last, my body, mind, and soul were nourished. Now I could look for pleasure in the inconsequential everyday things. I was waking up.

After almost three years of re-feeding my malnourished body and learning to trust the universe, I was just starting to distinguish between true hunger and anxiety. Anxiety was the need to feel different than I felt at that moment. Food was serving that need, momentarily.

I opened my journal to write about this.

I'm not hungry. I am. But I'm not. Perhaps it is better to say that the thing I used to know as hunger has left me. Underneath it there is a new feeling, something I am now able to name. That which I was calling hunger is truly anxiety.

For the next several months I was in significant pain. I could not walk, sit, or stand for more than five minutes, even lying down brought little relief. My normal lifestyle had completely changed due to this pain. Everything took longer to do, and many things I simply could not do. Even writing became difficult, as I could not stay in one position very long. Plus, the constant pain greatly stifled my creativity. What was left for me to do? Be.
Be? But what do you do with it?

Little by little I became aware of a sort of shifting in the fabric of who I had trained myself to become. As my injury persisted with little to no improvement and the months wore on, a different kind of wound was being healed. The injury I had lived with since childhood from the authoritative voices that told me happiness was found in accomplishments was subtly healing.

I was in the bathtub at 3:00 pm, again. It seemed to have become one of the most enjoyable parts of my day. Since my back injury, I had taken to shaving in the tub because it hurt to bend over while standing. The hot water helped to soothe my aches. At first, I felt guilty about soaking in the tub while there was still daylight left to be "productive". But then I realized that I was already living a dream life; I had enough money, I had spent the day with a friend at the beach, and my kitchen was stocked with healthy foods. The only thing left to "do" was to enjoy more fully what I already had, by doing things like soaking in a bathtub in the middle of the day.

It occurred to me that I was shaving my legs with a smile on my face. I hate shaving my legs, a task I've been cursed to perform daily since I was nine years old.

I laid there with the water still running. I felt the warm water cascade over my sore muscles, the soft glide of the razor, and the silky smooth skin. *This is what it feels like to be present. This is what it feels like not to run away from my body.* The thought was so simple, but it struck me like a slap in the face.

And then I saw my thighs, soft and plump. Months without exercise had left them atrophied, and years of emotional eating had covered them in a thick layer of stored emotions we call fat. I lovingly grabbed a handful on either side. *Oh, my dear thighs, you hold so much for me. Every emotion I've ever eaten lives right here, beneath my dimpled skin. You poor, beautiful thighs. I'm so sorry I've hated you for so long. You've carried me so far. I've run from every emotion and you've kindly stored them here for when I'm strong enough to deal with them. I guess now is that time.*

The tears I cried went unnoticed as falling water carried them away. Lightness filled my body. My guess is that several minutes passed before I became aware that I was still in the tub, laying with my hands on my belly, watching the rise and fall of deep belly breathing.

Months had passed and still, the pain persisted. I would start to feel better, start to hope, and then the slightest movement would send me back to square one. I still could not walk, sit or stand for more than a few minutes at a time. Being forced to spend so much of my day with myself, experiencing fully the pain in my body was the most wonderful thing that had ever happened to me. Everything took on new meaning because it had to. I sought satisfaction and pleasure in the smallest details of my day because, if not, I was left with only pain. As I began to purposely deepen my awareness of the present moment as my only source of pain relief, I also began to see beyond what I previously assumed was all there was to reality. It was almost as if I was looking into a hidden dimension. Suddenly a world of intuition, synchronicities, and deep knowing became a new reality for me.

The brilliant sun was almost too much goodness to bear. I lay sprawled on my towel, clutching an unopened library book. I watched a set of waves roll into the spot where the surfers had stationed themselves above the reef, 200 yards from shore.

The soundless wave rolled, towering higher until it threatened to topple. White foam crowned the crest. And then, just as the lip began to pitch forward, a surfer took his final paddle before leaping to his feet, in perfect synchronicity with the wave. He became one with the motion of the wave, and I became one with the entire scene. All anxiety was purged from my body. Thoughts became knowing, words had no place. I was in a meditative state I hadn't known was possible. Time dropped away. And so did my body.

Suddenly, my heart stopped beating. The scene in front of my eyes disappeared. Entirely out of nowhere, I was transported to a beautiful bed, surrounded by flowers, an ocean-facing window to my left. It was completely real, as real as the sand I had been laying on a moment before. Light poured in through the window. A man with strong eyes stood in front of the window. His hand reached down to hold mine as I laid in the bed. My hair was long, deep chocolate brown and falling around my face. Perhaps I had refused the chemo? I looked beautiful. I looked young. Maybe mid-forties. I held his hand, but neither of us held back our tears. No words were spoken. Goodbyes were exchanged through our fingertips. And then I closed my eyes. For good.

Laying there on the beach, the scene returned to normal. There were the surfers and the waves, here was the sand. But I felt different. I realized that, statistically, this crystal clear vision of my own death was more likely to become reality than not. Up until that point, I had never considered myself a woo-woo, hippy-dippy kind of person. I studied math and physics, and I still considered myself a scientist. But within me, a connection was forming to a current of energy that ran through me, and through everything else. I was beginning to see that I was part of a divine orchestra. I had always been playing my own music, but it felt a lot better if I joined in with the melody of the music that was already being played all around me.

Alone at home, I got up from my writing to walk to the kitchen for some water. I glanced down and noticed something out of place in the middle of the floor. I bent to pick up the foreign object, wondering where it had come from. It was a yellow-hued crystal. It was very warm and seemed to buzz slightly. I considered myself crazy for feeling such things from a random rock in the middle of my floor while I was home, alone.

Something told me to place the crystal on my lower back. It can't hurt, right? So I did. Immediately, something moved. There was a pulling and tugging sensation, and my pain lessened. It was tangible and significant, not imaginary. It happened.

Insanely curious and weirded out, I researched the crystal online. It turned out to be yellow quartz, known for physical healing properties. Like I said, I'm not a woo-woo person. But something was happening to me which I couldn't explain. Perhaps something had been happening to me all along, and I was finally letting it happen.

Suffering can be one of the quickest ways to return to knowing who we really are. Those who never suffer, who pad their lives with insurance policies, who are born into privilege, who never dare to live, who escape the full weight of negative emotions by using substances...these people may never wake up.

My back injury had become acute. The message from the universe was clear: stop and listen. I took time to rest. After three months without much exercise, I stepped on the scale. I saw a number I had never seen. It was a big number, ending in a zero. I had never been so heavy in my life, and with the least amount of muscle I had ever had. My legs had more cellulite than ever. Everything jiggled. Even as I write this, I recall the feeling powerfully. My eyes are pooling, my face is puckering, and my jaw is chattering against tears.

I was truly baffled. I had come so far in treating my body with kindness. I'd been honoring my hunger. I was eating mindfully. I wasn't eating from anxiety nearly as much.

Wasn't my body supposed to direct me to a healthier weight? I was listening to my body in new and profound ways. I was honoring all my body signals.

Yet, my body was getting fatter. Why would she do this? Why would she betray me in this way? I tried so hard to listen and respond with kindness, but she continued to throw my efforts in my face, causing me pain. I felt ripped off. Profound sadness filled me. I felt hopeless, cursed, flawed. I can't have what I want. I will never be a professional athlete. Why would the universe do this to me when I've done nothing but listen and respond to what I'm being told? It's not fair!

I went to the bathroom. As I sat there, my hands automatically grabbed the rolls forming on my stomach. They were new, and my body was having a hard time making sense of them. My body said to itself, "This is so fucking disgusting." I noticed a reaction to this thought. I took two deep breaths and moved closer to explore this reaction. My chest felt like it wanted to cave in. I dug my nails slightly into my skin, unconsciously trying to hurt my disgusting body.

I was playing a victim and I was aware of it. I reminded myself that nothing was happening *to* me. *I am a witness to what is happening within a body named Natasha. That body feels sad and hopeless. And I experience the body.* The harshness of the feeling dissipated quickly. The feeling itself remained, but the suffering from the feeling faded.

I had wished the healing process to take place all at once. The truth was that it had not. But something had changed. In the past, I had been sad and hopeless. In my new reality, I *experienced* sadness and hopelessness. And I tried my best to welcome them.

I reminded myself that I had to continue to believe that my

body was connected to a source of wisdom greater than myself. I had been holding onto the belief that my body would return to thinness after I had healed my relationship with food. I felt like I now had a better relationship with food than at any time since I was 10 years old. Yet, I was at my heaviest ever. *Maybe I am best in a heavier body.* The thought was crushing. It felt like my ribs were being compressed. My breathing grew labored and tears formed pools in my eyes. *Maybe I'll always be a double- digit dress size. That means my surfing will be limited, or at least different. Maybe I'll continue to gain weight as I age, like most people do.* These thoughts brought on a sweet mourning. Tears and sadness were appropriate. I appreciated them as I began to let go of the idea of a small body. And, as I let go of the thoughts, I released a tiny bit of the struggle. There was a little less fight in my life, a little more peace, a little less suffering.

Chapter 35: Sensual Healing

The awakening process was doing its work within me. I still needed an income. I returned to doing massage slowly. As my soul was opening within me, my bodyworks with my clients started to take on a whole new feel. I was able to drop the role of "sexy Katie" and just be my genuine self with my clients. The shame I felt around what I was doing began to ease and with this easy feeling came more clients who truly needed my help.

I began to feel things in people's bodies, non-physical things. Anger, for example, feels like dense body armor, under the skin but above the muscle. Angry people need elbows and body weight to break up their armor before the muscles can really be felt. It's almost as if I needed to be violent in order to access an angry person. Their anger keeps them separate and grants them an illusion of safety.

Fear lives in the glutes. It is the subtlest gripping, the flexing of the hamstring, the catching of the breath. One day, as I worked on a glute filled with fear, I gently coaxed out the tension. A pain shot through my own glute in the same spot I was touching on my client. Coincidence? Later in the massage, my heart started racing for no reason. I took a slow, steady, deep breath. The man did the same. After the massage, he informed me that he'd undergone a heart operation which made his heart beat faster than it should. He was often overtaken by waves of panic.

Anxiety makes muscles stringy. Sadness turns the body to mush. How did I know this? I don't know. Suddenly, I just did.

Men with otherwise impermeable exteriors lay naked and vulnerable in front of me, opening themselves for healing they didn't even know they wanted but desperately needed. I saw myself as a massage therapist who offered healing sensual touch, rather than something secretive or dirty. I was able to provide my clients with an energy release they could not experience in traditional massage. It felt very different than making myself into a sex object or doing work I didn't want to do simply because I needed the money. For the first time, I started to feel pride rather than shame, in the work I was doing. I felt more aligned with my true purpose than I had when I taught yoga or math. I could see my unique abilities manifested in a way that brought healing and light. The more I enjoyed my work, treating it like a meditation, the more connection I felt to clients' bodies. The more I connected, the more good I was able to do. And the more good I did, the more satisfaction I took in my work. I was in a beautiful upcycle.

The universe was sending me the perfect clients. Or, by knowing exactly what I enjoyed doing and where my boundaries were, I was attracting the perfect clients. I was given nothing but respect and appreciation. Fewer men pushed my boundaries or tried to get all they could from me, bartering for what they wanted from me like a used car sale. Instead, they were incredibly grateful to be able to bring me money in exchange for my services. It was almost as if the more I saw my own worth, the more worth I created. Even though I was working less due to my injury, somehow I was making more money.

I had slept with a lot of guys in the years following my second divorce. I have no desire to count. I'm sure I couldn't remember all of them if I tried. And since I knew I didn't actually want to make any of them a partner, I stopped dating them altogether and just skipped straight to the sex. All I had wanted was to feel powerful. But after my injury, I simply hadn't wanted to be with anyone. Rather, I wanted to be with the *right* one. I was tired of getting a poor night's sleep, a person I hardly knew lying next to me. I was tired of being ogled in the grocery store. I was weary of the constant text messages that came after a one night stand--wanting something from me, "Can I get a pic?" or "Let's trade massage." *Trade massage? Are you kidding me? Do you have any idea what my hourly rate for massage is? I could hire a professional to massage me for three times as long as what you will give me, and then you are gonna want* sex *from me, for free! No way.* My worth was loud and clear in my head.

Clients were offering to pay to massage *me.* They offered me numbers in the thousands for sex, and if I wasn't into it, I was turning them down. I was finally coming to know my worth and understanding that plenty of money will always be there. The pleasure of my company alone was worth good money. I wasn't going to give that away just for the satisfaction of knowing I was liked or attractive. For the first time ever I genuinely liked myself. I found myself attractive, even at my heaviest weight ever. I never thought I would know the freedom of not needing others approval but I was starting to taste it. All along I thought I needed a man for validation and financial security. It turns out I just needed to believe I was valid and my finances solved themselves. I was finding power within myself rather than putting it in the hands of others. Guys offered to take me out, but my response became, "Thank you, I'm flattered, but I'm just cruising right now. I'm not really doing the dating thing." I didn't need them. I didn't care if I hurt their egos by turning them down. It was so freeing. It would take someone really, truly special to be worth my time. I had never before felt this desire to be with just one person. Never, not even during my marriages. And all of this confidence was rising even as the number I saw daily on the scale slowly rose too.

My work became a source of daily satisfaction. I could see the good I was doing on the faces of my clients.

Dale came to see me every other week. He was happily married, a father of two. Dale's wife didn't get excited about sex. Dale craved a little excitement. He didn't want a new relationship; he loved his wife. So a girlfriend was out of the question. But his needs were real. So he and his wife made an agreement: do what you want, just don't throw it in my face, don't get emotionally involved, and be safe. Dale considered his visits with me part of maintaining a healthy lifestyle and healthy marriage. And I took satisfaction in being able to provide a hard to find service that was safe, discreet, professional, and filled with the compassion Dale desperately needed.

Jack was also a regular client. Well into his seventies, Jack spent much of his free time with a lot of female friends. Jack's friends were just friends. He loved being around their female energy. He enjoyed spending money on them, taking them sailing, and to fancy dinners. But Jack was old and set in his ways. He loved going home alone and arranging his days according to his own preferences. He simply needed a little sensual stimulation now and then. But stimulation from just anybody would not cut it, he needed someone to talk to, someone who could listen and offer compassion. I always had fun with Jack and he always compensated me generously.

Shawn, Cory, Daniel, and Josh were in their twenties and thirties. They were all handsome and had no problem meeting women. They were military guys, constantly on the move, and not interested in settling down. They were not at a point where they wanted a committed relationship. They were also not interested in getting their phones blown up by the emotional needs of the girls they met on Tinder. They didn't want to spend hours on dates hoping to get lucky, then hoping the girls would never call them back. They didn't want to sleep with drunk women they picked up in bars. But they did want the pleasure of being touched by a beautiful woman. To these guys I was the girl next door, hot, available, down to earth and relatable, yet posed no threat to their way of life. My services were a necessary part of their healthy sex lives.

Tim had been married for 28 years. He loved pleasing his wife. Generally, his wife did not reciprocate. He had expressed his desires. She was simply caught up in her own selfishness. He was thinking of making a change. He was starting to understand that maybe he deserved more. He wanted to treat himself to some self-care, to see how it made him feel. Tim's wife had no idea he was seeing me. I encouraged him to be honest with his wife. After several sessions, he said he had indeed spoken to his wife about his sexual desires and the conversation went far better than expected. It opened up a dialog about many issues in the marriage outside of the bedroom. Both parties agreed changes had to be made. Tim stopped seeing me after that.

Mike was born with a heart condition that gave him panic attacks if he got too worked up. This made sexual stimulation a very touchy situation. Mike didn't have a committed partner. But he couldn't have sex with someone who may not be sensitive to his needs. He was scared to become aroused and needed special handling. I was honored that he would trust me with his heart. Using breath work and eye contact, we worked through his racing heart rate. Several times, we had to ease off. I kept reassuring him that there was no end goal in mind. Simply relaxing and breathing through something scary was good enough. Mike left a much more confident man than when he arrived.

Jeremy had just gotten a divorce. He hadn't been touched by another woman in 18 years. He was nervous to get back out there. He wanted a safe place to experience his own emotions at being touched by a woman, without risking the emotional well-being of a new partner.

Todd and his wife had agreed to experiment sexually outside of monogamy. But Todd really didn't want to invest his time and emotions in a girlfriend. He just wanted to experience a rush that he hadn't felt in years, without bringing another person's emotions into his life.

Steve worked 70-80 hour weeks. He loved his job and he was good at it. There was no time nor desire in Steve's life for a girlfriend. But that didn't mean his urges were gone. The release and companionship he found with me allowed him more focus and clarity while at work.

Matt was a bundle of energy. Like a big Hawaiian teddy bear, he cracked jokes for the first 15 minutes of the massage. He cracked me up with his pidgin English:

"Yeah, when I go to make one nut I get a pinchin in my ball and a pain shootin' down da foot. Dat's why I came see you. Someone at home don't know I'm here, yeah? It make it kinda hard da blow one load ya know?"

"Yeah that would be hard," I offered. "Your body gets nervous because it senses something isn't right once it feels pain, so it won't let you cum. That can be hard on a woman's self-esteem. She might think she's doing something wrong."

"Exactly, Sistah, you know it!"

I thought of several possible contributors to Matt's foot pain. His glute was locked up and likely pressing on his sciatic nerve. The flexing of his body under the strain of thrusting during sex would likely to exasperate the nerve pressure. I also noticed that he had edema around his knees and ankles where fluid was pooling. Matt appeared to have circulation issues. It made perfect sense that he would feel like his blood supply was getting cut off. Acquiring and maintaining an erection requires a tremendous amount of blood, and his heart was having trouble keeping up.

During the massage, I focused on increasing circulation with long, sweeping, full-body strokes toward the heart. I used my hands and my bare upper torso to move heartward along the backs of his legs. I rolled Matt over and spent a significant amount of time massaging his groin area. In case anything was pinched, I wanted to relax the area completely. Then I began to work on the base of the penis, from the underside of the ball sack. Matt's eyes rolled back in his head as he let out a soft, "Whoa."

After several minutes of massaging around the penis, I reached for more oil and started to massage the shaft itself. Matt took in a deep breath.

"That's crazy, I've never felt anything like that!"

"It doesn't hurt does it?" I double-checked.

"No way, it's unreal!"

"Good. But please stop me if anything hurts." After the massage, Matt reported that nothing hurt and he hadn't felt that relaxed in months. I encouraged him, now that he knew he needed more time to relax before direct genital stimulation, to go home and talk with his wife about the best way to help him through what was going on in his physical body.

Kent had me laughing before I ever met him. At 62, his career as a former professional athlete had left his body a wreck. A nasty divorce 10 years earlier had left his heart a wreck, to boot.

We chatted casually for the first half of the massage. It turned out he coached in the semi-pro league I used to play in. We chatted about things we had in common, like sports injuries and how much we hated online dating.

I asked Kent why he hadn't dated since his wife left him. He described how much she'd hurt him. He said he preferred dating for only an hour or two at a time. He explained that a massage costs about the same as a date, and he was much more likely to leave feeling satisfied. I said that made sense. He said he generally didn't like to be touched. He admitted that it made him feel too much. I told him that it was brave of him to allow himself to be touched by me.

Kent revealed that a loving touch would overwhelm him with emotion, and possibly cause him to cry. But he quickly added that he would shut off the tears if they came. Through laughter, I reassured him that his tears would be a badge of honor for me. Then, more sincerely, I uttered,

"Let it flow if it flows, babe."

To shut off tears is to shut down emotions. It stops the flow of energy. Sexual stimulation is a flow of energy. You can be sexually aroused without emotion, but the arousal is far less powerful. The orgasm will feel cheap and unfulfilling. Like having a cup of noodles for dinner when you really wanted steak--it fills the belly but it doesn't feed the soul. To me, any emotion in a sexual encounter is good.

Soon, we fell silent. I touched his body with a single intention: find the pain and pull it out.

As we neared the final moment of the massage, Kent gripped my shoulder with one hand and, with the other, held my face. His eyes locked on mine. It was intense. I wanted to look away, but I knew the human connection was what Kent

needed the most.
Kent had his finish and tears did indeed wet his eyes. He dropped my hand to wipe them. I put my hand over his heart and counted three deep breaths. Then I told him simply to take his time and enjoy every sensation in his body.

I'd arrived at a whole new understanding of human sexuality. The movement of stagnated sexual energy is a need. If energy backs up anywhere in the body, blockages occur and physical and psychological distress result. Sometimes professional help is needed to move stagnation. Sexually, this is where some people may turn to affairs, emotional shutdowns, angry outbursts, substance abuse, and a whole host of darker sexual expression. Down the road, this leads to sexual dysfunction and emotional death. Even farther down the road are the physical issues that come from being cut off from one's emotions. Sexual release is a hunger that should not be ignored. There is some virtue in restraint, to be sure. Just as stealing food that does not belong to you, or anxiously overindulging can have devastating consequences. Going without food for long periods is possible, and can also be very healthy. Both science and ancient cultural practices support the value of fasting. But starvation is real. Eventually, the body will wither and die if it is not fed. Chronic undereating, overeating, and eating food with little nutritional value, causes suboptimal health. For the highest quality of life, we must balance how much we feed our hunger and the things we feed it. All these dynamics applied to sexuality. My work was to offer an option for nourishment. But not just cheap, drive-thru calories. My goal was to offer something that fed the mind, body, and soul. It was up to the client to use it responsibly. Some of them ate slowly, chewing every bite, taking it all in. Some of them gulped it down, paid their tab, and walked out immediately forgetting what they had for lunch.

Food, comfort, pleasure, addiction, sex, love. I was just beginning to understand how related these were. When I didn't feel loved, I wanted to eat. When I wanted to make someone feel loved, I offered them food. When I was horny, I wasn't hungry. When men came to see me, they wanted much more than sexual release. They wanted to be cared for. They wanted love. Sometimes my clients felt more love and compassion with me than they had felt in years with their actual partner. And, sometimes, I connected better with clients who never touched me than I had with guys I'd slept with.

I started baking cookies for my clients. My mom's famous monster cookies, to be specific. I can count on one hand the number of times my mom has said "I love you". But there is no counting how many of her monster cookies I've eaten. And that's why I gave these cookies to my clients. It was a way of saying, "I see you. You matter." To me, cookies are little circles of love.

Chapter 36: Ready for Love

Alongside the pride I now took in my work, a new space opened up within me. I saw the power of sexuality for what it was. It was no longer a way of gaining validation. It was a healing and life- changing gift that I could choose to use for others or for myself. I became more and more stingy with my arousal when working on my clients. I took great compassion for them, I gained pleasure from seeing the rewards of my healing work all over their faces, but I stopped allowing my own sexuality to be awakened. I wanted to reserve my sacred sexuality for one person, more deserving than all the rest. I wanted to be with someone who I trusted. Sexual arousal is an exchange of energies. If I let myself become aroused with someone, I needed to be able to trust I was not inviting negativity or darkness inside me. I didn't want to ever have to tell someone no again. I wanted the next person I opened sexually toward to be so attentive to my experience that my comfort zone was never pushed to the point where "no" was necessary. I didn't mind touching and stimulating my clients, but when they wanted to stimulate me in return, I drew a firm line. I wanted one person to love me so deeply that I yielded everything to him or her. It wasn't a hunger or an urge, but simply an open space quietly waiting to be filled.

One afternoon, aided by plant medicine, I became lost in deep meditation. I gazed at the clouds and everything was so vibrant. I could see how connected everything was. My breath, the trees, the spinning of the planet. My life seemed so full. For a brief moment, I knew deep in my being how loved I was, how worthy of love I was, how much love I had to give. The clouds seemed to play a symphony in the sky, rapturous and fluid. The music of life itself. The symphony seemed to say that the most beautiful parts of life were those I had overlooked while working too hard to accomplish something.

I watched the symphonic clouds for hours that afternoon, entranced by their music. After the meditation, I knew I needed more moments of such beauty. I knew they were possible without any substance in my system. *I'd love to go to the symphony sometime soon,* I thought to myself. After that meditation, something in my physical body that had been broken for a very long time resumed working again. I could feel the hormones that regulate hunger, after years of being out of balance, had once again come into alignment.

That very same afternoon, my appetite for food stopped. For the first time in memory (except maybe when I had the flu), food didn't sound good. Around 8:00 pm, after not having eaten since breakfast, I made a bowl of rice and steamed broccoli. It was the most satisfying meal I had eaten in months. The next morning, after a solid night's sleep, food still didn't sound good. Around noon, I made a smoothie. It was 8:00 pm before I felt like eating again. Only rice and broccoli sounded good. The next several days were the same story. Seven pounds fell off during that week. Another ten pounds would follow, more slowly. I had never lost weight without trying. Eventually, my appetite came back, but not before twenty pounds were gone for good.

My anxiety had melted away along with my appetite. For the first time, I experienced the richness and depth of ordinary things. I wasn't hungry, because I was already full. I was full of the everyday pleasures of living life. And my body realized it would be okay without a meal every three hours. Eating disorder literature describes that every year of active disorder requires one half to a full year of recovery for the body to feel safe again. I had been actively restricting calories for at least ten years. It had been five years since I first admitted I had a problem.

A few days after the symphony of the clouds, shortly after my appetite had died, I went to watch the sunset at the beach. The same guy who had told me my body looked so good at its fastest a couple months back, again approached me. Making no small talk, he got right to the point:

"I was wondering if you'd like to go to the symphony with me this weekend."

I was used to turning guys down when they asked me out. I could see they didn't want a date but they did want sex. But before he'd gotten all the words out of his mouth, I blurted, "Yes, my answer is yes!" I knew this was different. I knew that the clouds had sent this person to take me to hear the actual symphony. But I had no idea the many other reasons our fateful meeting had been arraigned in the heavens.

We talked non-stop during the hour and a half drive to the Honolulu Symphony Orchestra. We didn't mention the weather, aside from a discussion of climate change and the role of the Average Joe in creating change for a sustainable future. The topics ranged from choosing your attitude when facing adversity, to the goodness in each one of us, to the unity of all things, to the existence of all inside a consciousness of one.

I hadn't known that a human like this one existed. A massive fan of women, he said they should be running the world. He had a superhuman ability to draw forth a smile from anyone he encountered. Always cracking a joke, never impatient, he was in a constant state of awakening to what was going on around him. He used words I didn't know and gently challenged me when my thinking was small. He had a real job where he made real money. No messy divorces complicated his history. He had abandoned no children to roam the earth, fatherless. He wanted to travel as much as possible, and his job allowed for it. Oh, and he was a boat captain, a surfboard maker, and a phenomenal surfer. He'd lived for years in the Caribbean, sailing boats and surfing. As a result, he had the most admirable "take it easy" vibe. The cherries on top were his coffee-colored skin, piercing eyes, and perfectly groomed beard.

I was hooked. The first night, he didn't touch me. A long line at the bathroom took me away from him for a time. When I returned, I passed a column of guys, all hunched over with their heads to their phones as they waited for their dates. But not him. He sat with perfect posture on a bench, a massive smile on his face, staring off into the crowd of people. When I asked him what he was looking at, he said he was looking at everything. When I asked him what made him smile, he said that I did, and so did everything else. When I asked him what he was thinking, he said he wasn't actively thinking anything, just watching his thoughts. When I asked him how long he had practiced meditation to enable him to be in such a state so quickly and easily, he said his whole life--and not really ever at all.

An hour into the second date, I let him know I was attracted to him. He giggled.

"Good, me too...I mean, I'm attracted to you, not me!"

Later that night, I found myself in my bed, lying underneath him, both of us trying to catch our breath. He asked me what I had to do the next day. I knew I had to tell him. I really liked this guy, but I also really liked my job. If he couldn't be okay with it, then he wasn't right for me. I wasn't going to hide who and what I was in order to get this man to like me. I took a deep breath. *Just say it, Natasha. If he doesn't like it, then he can go on his way!*

"So..." I paused, "I do sensual massage."

"Okay," was all he said.

"And, I mean, I love it. It makes me feel beautiful. It's fun, and I have the most amazing clients who really benefit from what I'm doing. Guys have sexual release who haven't been able to do that in years. Sometimes guys cry on my table. It's really an honor to do this kind of work. But I understand if you can't be with a girl who gives topless massage and touches men's naked bodies for a living."
"No, it's cool."

But the very next day, he stood me up. He called me an hour after he was supposed to meet me, explaining that he had been stuck at work and wasn't able to step away to call me. He needed to work late and was canceling on me. My anxiety was overwhelming. Guilt and shame flooded back. *No, Natasha, this is a man who can be trusted. When he says something, he means it. Try believing that, just try!*

Two days later, I asked him point blank, "Do you mind my work? I get the feeling that you don't like it."

"What? Do I hear guilt behind that statement?" he questioned me. "What you do is saintly... saintly." He emphasized it twice. "That is important work and incredibly difficult." He was totally serious. He added, "And I think it's so hot!"

"Nat," he continued, "I'm the type of person who says exactly what I think. If I say something, I mean it. You can believe that. If I am here with you, it is because I want to be. I only do what I want to be doing. You can try trusting that and see how you go."

I believed him. He was committed to being himself, to his own uncompromising happiness. And I felt unconditional permission to be who I was, too. A permission I had never before been granted.

Chapter 37: Relationships are Not My Strong Suit

Everything about our relationship was like a fairytale. He fell all over himself to take care of me, jumping at my every need. He adored my body, constantly telling me and touching me. He was hilarious and made me laugh exactly when I needed to. My body felt pain-free for the first time in five months.

But anxiety and insecurity seemed prerequisites for any of my relationships. They soon found their way into this one. I thought I had awoken, I had changed! But correcting old patterns takes diligence and daily mindfulness.
I am guilty of losing myself in every relationship because I'm afraid that doing what I really want, being authentically myself, will make me a burden. It plays out in simple things, starting with food. I don't eat what I want because I'm eating with him. I don't eat as much as I want because I feel that I should eat less than him, I don't eat when I want because if I bring out the snacks at 9:00 pm, I'm afraid he'll think I'm a big fatty. A woman's needs always come second to those of her family, after all. This pattern of behavior chips away at me, separating me from my desires, I am unable to speak up for what I want.

My speaking up would, in fact, inconvenience my partner. Relationships are inconvenient. But I don't feel worthy of being an inconvenience. Instead, I stay up later than I want because he wants to stay up. I drink because he is drinking. I put up with dishes left in the sink that bug me and sock left on the floor. I watch TV that drives me nuts because he is watching it. But I can't say anything because I'm afraid he won't like me if I prioritize my desires.

I'm far less productive than I would be on my own, and that gives me anxiety. We lay around all morning, naked in bed, and he keeps wanting to cuddle--and I keep thinking of all the stuff I like to do that I'm not doing because he wants snuggle time. The house needs to be cleaned. I haven't written anything in days. I'd love to go for a swim. Instead, I just lay there, my heart racing from anxiety. I assume that if I get out of bed, put on my clothes, and fetch my laptop or the vacuum, then he will be offended. Or, if I ever do get that far, I cut my work time short because I feel rude that he's lying there in the bed while I'm over here clicking away at my keyboard.

My relationships have been ruled by shoulds. I should spend time with him. I shouldn't make special requests. I should suck his dick. I should cook him something he likes for dinner because if I don't, he might leave. One of us is going to have to compromise. Or one of us is going to have to say "I'm sorry, but this just isn't working for me." Do I know where I stand? Do I know how much compromise I can make? I know he will walk away if he feels he cannot be authentic to himself. The question is, will I?

And if I won't, then he holds all the power and I start to lose myself. I know he won't fundamentally change who he is. He told me, "What you see is what you get." And I don't want him to change. I fell in love with who he is. To change would diminish him. And he feels the same about me. So, if our lifestyles conflict, will I settle for less than the joy I had being single, simply because I don't want to hurt him?

A couple of months into our relationship my back started aching again. My appetite came back, strong. Being stuck in the house with limited mobility left me with nothing to do but think. Normally, I avoided my thoughts by staying busy, taking risks, and accomplishing things. My thoughts were going wild. Physically static, I remained very active in the brain. I wasn't relaxed, I was just immobile. *I thought I had found the perfect man and then he turned out to be a human, flaws and all. Go figure. Should I stay? Is he worth investing my time and energy? Is he holding me back from opportunities I could have if I was single? Could someone better for me be out there?*

In the midst of all that anxiety, I reinjured my back. I was just riding in the car on a bumpy road. One pothole too many, and I was in misery again, worse than the first injury. I was devastated. Six months of rest and PT, six months without surfing. Six months of laying around, fighting off my depression, and then--wham! Pain like I had never felt before. *Oh my god, I'm not going to get better! This pain is never going away. My life as a surfer and an athlete is over. This is what I will be for the rest of my life.*

I laid in bed, powerless under the excruciating pain. Getting injured was hard. Getting reinjured from doing nothing after six months of rest...that was a whole other level of hard. As it often does with chronic pain, depression set in. Along with it, even more anxiety. I sought a scapegoat for my misery. As a normal human, my new partner came with flaws, and these became my targets.

Each day, I spent at least 20 hours in bed, an ice pack on my back. And the days stretched into weeks. I suffocated in thought. *He's not the right man for you. He has no ambition in life. He doesn't support you like you need. You make more money than he does, and he has no retirement plan. What will you do when he is old? He drinks too much. He watches too much TV. He doesn't eat healthy. He smokes cigarettes.*

The truth was, he did have some issues. He had fallen into several low-energy habits, smoking, having a few beers every day, eating fast food, and watching a lot of TV. I knew he could be doing more with his life. I saw his potential so clearly. I also knew that I did not want to be with a man who wasn't physically healthy--and he wasn't. I wasn't going to try to change him. I had done that too many times, and I knew it never worked. So there it was. He was amazing, but he was limiting himself. I knew I had to stand up for what was best for me. I loved this man. But to tell him that his lifestyle didn't fit with mine felt the same as calling him a loser. Which I didn't believe was true. I was terrified that I might hurt him. I couldn't do it.

My thoughts raced through the days, into the nights, penetrating even my dreams. I fell further into depression than I had been in years. My body didn't work. My boyfriend was emotionally unavailable. Each day, he slipped deeper and deeper, further away from me and further into the TV. I wrote about the situation, then thought about it, then dreamt about it, then woke up thinking about it, over and over. I was losing it. Thoughts of suicide were daily on my mind.

Finally, I told him it wasn't working. I told him that the drinking, the smoking, the ordering pizzas and drive-through food, the TV watching, and never getting out of the house...well, it wasn't the lifestyle I wanted to live. All of it could have been said months earlier, plainly and matter of factly, had I the confidence to do so. Instead, powered by weeks of anxiously stewing on these facts it came out much more like an attack on his character.
Being the gracious, thoughtful man that he is, He considered the validity of my words. He said it wasn't how he wanted to live either. He said he wanted to change. It had never been important to him when he was younger but he knew it was important now. He would quit drinking and quit smoking and learn to eat healthier if I would show him. I wanted to believe him.

But just like all the rest, he didn't follow through. Well, he sorta did. After a few days, he cut back on the things he said he'd quit but it wasn't enough. He still smoked a few times per day, drinking went back to every other day and the TV still remained on for hours a day. I didn't believe his sincerity. I learned my lesson before. They either change or they don't. There is no use waiting around for them to get their shit together. They don't need to taper back. They need to quit. Behavioral change doesn't take time, you just walk up to the TV and turn it off. You don't crack another beer open. You don't go through the drive-through. *You simply don't stick your fingers down your throat --or wait, maybe it's more complicated than that--nevermind, that's totally different.*

I wasn't giving out any second chances this time. I had been with too many addicts and my heart could not take another round of that kind of beating. After three weeks of sitting back and watching, I exploded on him.

"I just don't feel like you're following through. Your unhealthy behavior is affecting our sex life. You sit around watching TV and drinking beer and you have no drive in life or in bed. I miss getting the shit rammed out of me! You don't want me, you don't burn for me. You don't burn for anything. You just exist."

"Well, change takes time, as you know, because you have had your share of growth in your life. And as far as the fucking, I'm not that guy. That's just not my style," was his response.

No. I had been hurt one too many times by guys using substances, promising to change. He was saying all the same things they had said. I wasn't putting myself through that bullshit again. So I left.

I hadn't been much out of bed in over a month. With my back

as awful as it was, I had no idea how I would make the trip or how I would take care of myself. But I booked a ticket to Mexico anyway.

The instant I got back to my Mexican apartment, all my anxiety and depression fell away and my back felt better. I was once again living beachfront and taking time to go lay on the beach every morning, even swimming if I felt up for it. I would spend an hour or two in meditation daily. No more thoughts, just stillness. But almost as soon as I felt better and the anxious thoughts trickled away, I missed him.

I missed sharing life experiences with a partner. Of course, all the guys in the little Mexican town whom I had known previously were thrilled that I was back. But I wasn't interested. I wanted just one person. I knew who he could be if he just dropped his bad habits. And I desperately wanted that guy back. But the same could be said of either of my ex-husbands.

In Hawaii, we had lived on a cul de sac in suburbia, twenty minutes from the nearest beach. After having left him I was back at the ocean, swinging in a hammock in the shade, spending a couple of hours in the sunshine each day. My thoughts began to slow. In a few days, my eyes began to open. Most of my depression had nothing to do with him. My thoughts were getting the best of me. My incessant overthinking caused my suffering. Yes, change was needed, but suffering was a choice. I blamed my insecurities on his sex drive. Also, lack of access to nature had been crushing me. Back at the beach, it was much easier to control my thinking. After two weeks, I called him, just to see how he was. His response shocked me.

"I have neither smoked nor drank since you left. You were right. It wasn't healthy and I can do better."

I wanted to see him. But I was scared he would just let me down again, like all the rest.

Chapter 38: The Journey

At 4:00 am on a Friday[E2] , I hailed a taxi heading south down Mex-200. My phone in one hand, I carried a beach umbrella in the other and a pack on my back. I slipped into the cab. I texted my friend, Abi, to let her know to come outside to meet us. *Shit, I forgot my phone isn't getting data service.* I had been on a WiFi call with Sprint for hours the previous week, trying to connect my phone to local Mexican towers, but no one could help me. The internet comes and goes in Puerto, part of the flow of life there. The previous night, the WiFi came back up and I was able to get back on WhatsApp to organize today's adventure.

I dropped all my things into the back of the taxi. When we reached Abi's house, I jumped out to whistle for her in classic Mexican style. Who needs a working phone? Minutes later, the driver dropped us off at the base of a dark hiking trail. As the taxi pulled away, I rummaged in my pack for my brand new iPhone, to use its flashlight. The iPhone wasn't there. It wasn't anywhere. A sinking feeling grabbed my stomach. I knew exactly where it was. I could almost picture it, speeding away in the back of that taxi. Nevermind. I had bigger fish to fry. The last thing I wanted to do was bring bad vibes into what was about to go down.

After a short walk, we arrived at a secluded beach. A trillion stars glimmered. Heat lightning struck on the horizon. Multiple shooting stars raced across the sky with every minute. How lucky! We had timed this voyage for the week of an annual meteor shower.

We laid out towels on the sand. I produced a small bottle filled with a dark, sweet-smelling liquid, prepared for me by a shaman. Two months earlier the shaman had read energy and

prescribed a daily dose of herbs to cleanse me in preparation for today's event. I had eliminated all low energy substances from my life - coffee, alcohol, weed, tobacco, and even my relationship that wasn't vibrating at it's highest. My system was now considered pure enough to handle the spiritual awakening that this little bottle would catalyze.
"May you show me all that I need to see. May I be receptive? May I allow your healing work to be done in me without restriction." I prayed aloud, then gulped the liquid.

And then, we waited. Soon, the offshore winds picked up as cool air raced down from the mountains. We shivered, backs pressed against the cool sand. We put on all the clothes we'd brought with us and huddled together. My back ached, with no padding against the hard- packed sand of the beach. Wanting to stay near Abi's warmth, I resisted movement, which made the aching worse. An hour passed as streaks of light from all directions filled the sky.

What I clearly remember is that nothing changed. I didn't feel stoned or drunk or high. But my eyes opened to a spectrum or reality just beyond visible light. I wasn't making it up. I was simply able to see it for the first time. I saw beautiful neon pinks, purples, blues, and greens, like the weaving of an Aztec blanket. The colors filled the sky, forming vibrant geometric patterns. Otherwise, I felt fully normal. Except for the pain in my back, which I could now feel in a very different way. It was a black, swirling vortex, spinning like a galaxy. It flung dark, purple-tinged tentacles around my body. The more I focused on the vortex, the more I could feel its movements. It radiated, hot and alive. It hooked itself into my tailbone, sacrum, and lower back. The ball of pain moved as the earth beneath me also moved. I sensed the movement of the ocean under me. The waves at the beach that morning were massive. Rip currents ran quick along the shore break and under the sand. I felt the rips through the beach, and the dark energy in my back moved with them. Sucked one direction and then the other.

The energy wanted to descend into the ground. With each revolution, the terrible black and neon purple ball in by back flung a tentacle from its outer edge. The tentacle of pain moved through my body, crackling through energy meridians. Like lightning, the energy sought grounding. With each crack, it connected to the earth underneath me. Having found its path, the energy bled out of me and into the beach.

So that was it. The pain in my back and tailbone wasn't anything more than energy looking to be released. I could see it clearly now, twenty minutes into my journey. I was holding on to the energy. In fact, I had invited it in and placed it there for storage. Strangely, the energy didn't seem evil, just stale and dead. It felt like blocked-up gunk that wanted to go back into the earth's core to be melted back into light. Like toxins filtered from the body to be defecated, the energy was simply a byproduct of living. But this particular ball of energy had become trapped, like a years-long constipation--years of anxiety, years of striving. All of nature conspired to extract the toxins from me. But I clung to the stale energy, like a pig wallowing in its own feces. How I hadn't seen this dynamic earlier, I don't know. It was all so clear. For years, I had been collecting this gunk and storing it in my lower back and hips, terrified to let it flow from me. It felt like greed, it felt like fear, it felt like worry, *What if I need this later? I simply can't let go. Letting go would make me vulnerable.* I failed to trust in the flow of the universe.

The first rays of light broke on the horizon. Bugs started buzzing. Their buzzes seemed to sing darkness out of me, and sing me into light. I felt the buzzes as pulses of energy, dislodging the entrenched energy. The ground slowly, gently pulled at the darkness. The pain of letting go was intense. My body ached so badly, I began to sob. My sinuses opened and mucus flowed. I cried harder. It felt good. The tears and snot felt like the blackness seeping out.

I felt bad leaving Abi alone in the cool dawn air, but my body craved the cold. The cold didn't feel good, but it felt healing. I rolled over, placing my entire body on the sand. I shivered and shook and the darkness bled from me. Flies landed on me and ate the darkness that seeped from my skin. This is what flies are for, I realized. They eat away the shit of life. I thought about the many dogs I'd encountered on Mexican beaches, lying in the sand, shivering the night away, bugs swarming their soft parts. The dogs know. I thought about the trees that rose behind me. I felt them shivering, too. Nature feels the cold and the sting of life, but it doesn't resist or pull away. It doesn't cling to what it doesn't need. Trees least of all, and they live to be hundreds of years old. Maybe humans could too, if we didn't resist the natural flow of purification, if we didn't cling to the past or fear the future. How many times had I retreated into myself to avoid the sting of cold and fly bites? How many lessons had I avoided learning because I was afraid? I was afraid of life. I saw it clearly. Afraid to be broke, afraid to be unique, afraid to have a voice, afraid to be big, afraid I wasn't big enough, afraid I would not have enough.

I saw and felt the flow of energy all around me, in the trees, in the bugs, in the air. It was an ocean aswirl in neon currents. It was a fabric from which everything was knit. Was this consciousness? Was this God? It was so clear, I was shocked that I had never seen it before. A wave of energy would rush in, bugs would buzz louder, a flock of birds would leave the roosts, and the darkness inside me would swirl wider. A breeze would wash in, more of the gunk would flow from me. It was so beautiful. All of nature flowed, each flow playing its part within an endless improvisation. It's why birds fly south.

It's why fish swim upstream. It's why we feel drowsy at night. It's why, in little Mexican villages, where people live closer to nature, without cell phones and freeways and shopping malls, they want for nothing. When they are hungry, food flows to them. When they need money, it arrives. These wise people hold loosely, to allow the flow to work. They rarely save money or stock up on food. To do so would block the flow. They have few possessions and feel welcome to the possessions of others. Sharing is a given.

It's why the internet comes and goes in Puerto. It's why I lost my phone when I was too attached to it. I was too attached to my Instagram stories and my followers. I was blocking life's vital forces, always striving for better photos of myself, more likes, more comments. *I can't fucking believe I just lost my brand new phone. Money and items and a master plan mean nothing, nothing.* More tears. Lots more tears.

The sun rose, bringing a bit of warmth. I stood, slowly. I stretched. Some of the darkness loosened from the stiff places where it had come to rest. It melted from me. But it stuck in my hip, where a remnant of the black ball still dwelled, swirling and pulsing. I shook my leg, attempting to displace the ball. I started to walk. Gravity sucked the black ball down my leg. I started to run. With each stride, the impact of my foot on the sand subtly broke up the darkness. But I was too weak and had to stop. I knelt in the sand and put my forehead on the beach, massaging my third eye back and forth, still crying.

A fisherman came by with his nets. He was the first human I had seen, besides Abi. He examined me. I was hunched over, squatting and drawing in the sand with a stick. I tried to look normal and offered a tiny wave. *Normal?* What if all of us were just who we are, and *normal* was never invented? I would be free to move how I wanted to move. My creativity and life force would flourish. Fuck being normal. Fuck what anyone thinks. I want to flow. Right now, my intuition tells me to be grounded, close to earth.

The trip was near to having run its course. My thoughts had become lightning clear. A new truth cemented itself in my mind. Nature flows. I must flow, too. I must stop clinging to money and safety. Nature is the answer. Living in harmony with nature means releasing energy. No wonder living on a cul de sac in a suburb in Hawaii, sitting in front of the TV, spending no time in nature, my energy had been so badly blocked that it balled up into a black vortex of pain. Substances that move us away from our truest selves also block energy. Alcohol, foods with bad karma, TV, electronics...oh my god, my phone! I did not want that shit. Of course, the flow of energy took it from me when I could not surrender it on my own. Everything that had ever been taken was taken by nature; I was never in control anyway. I could fight the flow. But I would always lose. The pain in my body was sure confirmation that my fighting had to end.

Suddenly, I could see everything for what it was. I began to have visions of things as if they were right in front of my eyes. I saw roaches crawling on all of that shit. I saw the ball of dark energy enlarge each time I engaged with worry, thoughts about the future, and self-promotion on Instagram. I saw my clinging to money as a lack of trust in the flow. The lack was a dark cloud of flies, swarming around me. I saw how money could be filled with light and energy, bouncing around from person to person, easily entering my hand and easily flowing from it. I saw crisp $100 bills, filled with potential for light and life, and I saw older, softer bills swarming with roaches and darkness from the negative energy they carried after long lives in circulation. I no longer wanted to hold on to money. I no longer needed a ten-year plan to feel safe. The flow would provide.

———

My mind shifted to the man I left him back in Hawaii, three weeks earlier. I wanted him back. He intuitively understood energy and flow and I could see that now. He felt all that I was just starting to see, and he had lived with that flow for his entire life. He had just the right amount of money, and as soon as he got too much, he easily let it go, giving it away or buying something he truly needed or taking a trip. I saw how he never forced decisions. He never thought about something before the time came to think about it. And when the time came to stop thinking, he would easily let it go. He hated his phone and driving. It pulled him away from flow.

But I could see how darkness hooked into him, too. I recalled the many days he lay on the couch, sunlight blocked from streaming in by drawn shades, the TV blaring some type of darkness. Little roaches crawled all over him, loving every minute of it. I remember pulling him into the light, literally grabbing his hand and begging him to take me outdoors. In those moments, I could see the darkness that covered him, resisting me. He had polluted his body with darkness, alcohol still filtering through his liver from days before, cigarette smoke clinging to his skin and mouth, toxic food blocking him from the inside out. I remember in those moments looking at him, feeling no sense of attraction, actually repelled by him. The roaches were crawling all over him too. I was in love with him; his blockages were what pushed me away.

I wanted to see him soon. But I knew that when I saw him next, he must be at his purest for I could have nothing but purity around me if I was going to release the black ball within me that manifested as back pain. To release the darkness, I must vibrate high.

It made sense that we had resisted each other sexually. A ball of darkness lived in my root chakra region. It made me clench my lady parts. That darkness would respond only to force. In order to penetrate that darkness, my orgasms had to be forced with power, speed, and strength. And he does not force, he flows. I could not relax to receive his gentle, flowing love. In return, he did not feel safe to open to me. Because I wasn't safe. And no wonder I resisted him, when I could taste and smell the darkness on his body. Those dark, crawly bugs from the TV were coming nowhere near my most delicate parts. If I was to heal my back and live to my potential, I could no longer have casual sex with low vibrational partners.

In my mind, I saw him at his purest and me at mine. I am flowing. My beautiful feminine energy is slow, graceful, illogical, creative, and vibrant, just like nature. My soul dances easily through life, with no need to control or conquer. His strong, steady, bold, and confident masculine energy is drawn out by the feminine in me. We draw each other. My soft exterior is easily penetrated by his firm pursuit. I am happy to receive his masculine energy into my body. As a result, my body gives birth to even more light, strong enough to build a human and bring it into this world.

I also saw my mom for what she is. A pure, innocent, sweet little girl. Darkness lived on her like that slimy, fat character from Star Wars. Just like me, years of the need to accomplish and achieve had blocked her own flow. Rolling layers of grey fat now covered the lovely innocence that still lived within her, languishing and forgotten. My mom knows all about flow and connection, but she's lost herself to the rules of her church and the opinions of others. At that moment I knew I could love her because I finally saw who she truly was.

The sun was getting hot. Abi was rousing. We went together for a dip in the ocean, giggling like little girls as each wave smacked us. "Would you be offended if I took my top off?" asked Abi.

"Not at all!"

We both swiped off our tops. We stood on the sand, facing the ocean, waves lapping at our feet. I felt energy being stripped from my naked breasts, flowing out in the sea breeze. A hot spot of dark energy pocked the lower outside edge of my right breast. This energy will turn cancerous, I could feel it unless I released it. It made sense that underwire bras cause breast cancer; they blocked the flow of energy. Of course, deodorant causes breast cancer; it prevents sweat and toxins from being released back to the flow as they need to be. All cancer is just blocked energy. Breasts are accumulations of life force. They are a woman's way of giving life to others. When they are restricted, life force becomes blocked and dead.

Stared out over the ocean, we let our bellies stick out. The receding tide seemed to pull on them.

"I've been sucking that thing in since I was 10," I told Abi, "No wonder energy is blocked in that area." As I let my belly go soft, the urge to vomit struck. I wanted all that blocked up gunk out of me. Instead, I got a case of the hiccups and, little by little, I burped it up.

We spent the next five hours laying on the sand, massaging our bellies with warm stones, letting the waves pummel us and coalesce with the flow of energy within our bodies.

"Do you think you can feel the pull of the tides in your body?" I asked Abi.

"Probably."

We tuned in, and both arrived at the same feeling: the tide was going out, but was on the verge of switching. We looked out over the ocean. Suddenly, it went flat. Double overhead sets fell to one-foot waves.

"Fancy a proper swim?" I asked Abi, mimicking her Welsh accent. The ocean had spoken to me. She was giving us a little window of opportunity to swim in deep water beyond the dumping waves of the shore break. If we swam out now, we would have plenty of time to enjoy some moderate exercise and still get back to the beach without risking powerful waves breaking on our heads.

The best surfers are those who feel the greatest connection to the ocean. They have a sixth sense about how the energy flows. They didn't learn how to surf intellectually. They feel which waves will open up to them. The best way to surf is to clear your mind of all agendas and let the natural rhythms dictate when you enter, and how long you stay. Surfing is tapping into the feminine. I've been forcing my surfing since trying to create an Instagram following from it, wanting to look cool, wanting recognition for how good I was surfing, wanting to conquer something. I've been striving and training, rather than flowing and enjoying. The way a surfer surfers always reflects the way she lives.

Recalling my lost phone, I laughed. How wonderful it felt to be disconnected. I didn't want it back. I wanted to disconnect from that dark energy and meld myself with the rhythms of nature. I laughed every time I saw Abi, in all her youthful innocence and perky little tits, bouncing around in the waves. She seemed to have gotten younger by ten years.

The rest of the morning flowed for us. With no phone, no place to be, and nothing to accomplish, we laid in the sand, walked the beach, stretched, moved to the shade, and then back to the ocean.

I realized that it is possible to feel this good every day. It is a very feminine way to feel, without tasks to accomplish. Tasks are masculine. I could even see myself with a baby, having no agenda in life but to be with my child and allowing its father, or even the flow of life itself, to care for our human needs. I saw us playing in the ocean together without a care for tasks or money- making. I've seen the indigenous people here in Mexico living this way. No real work is ever done, no one goes to a job. People fish and cook and garden and take naps and play with their children. It's not possible to live this way when you want things like Instagram followers and blog readers, a better car, a new iPhone, and new surfboards. But if you are happy with a simple dwelling and a few changes of clothing, you could feel amazing all day, every day.

But I cling to these other things, and now they have clung to me, a big black ball of stuck energy living in my back and hips. Of what good are a car and an iPhone if you are in chronic, severe pain?

Being a part of modern society limits our ability to flow with the rhythms of nature. Like clinging to a rock at the bottom of the river, the currents of life try to move us toward wellbeing. Worse, it is like swimming upstream against the current of happiness. The more we cling and strive, the more we resist the flow, the worse the pain of life stings. I have known this for some time, but on that day I literally felt it.

On our walk back, I was very fatigued. Just as I stopped to rest, a woman appeared on a bicycle cart, selling cold fruit water. Everything was flowing. The natural flow of the universe anticipates my needs and provides for them in the exact moment they arise. There is no need to worry, ever.

After this experience, I made two lists. One of the things I wanted to release, and another of the things I wanted to increase.

To Release:
- Saving money and things for the future "just in case".
- Using technology. Spending so much time on the internet trying to get publicity in order to make money. Stopping this would mean letting go of making a name for myself, which has been a blockage for my entire life. Accomplishments and achievements no longer serve me.
- Relationships that do not bring light.
- Strict schedules which encourage productivity and accomplishment but limit the flow of energy
- Eating when I don't really need to eat. Food exists to bring light, but nature also brings light. Sometimes I want to eat when there are other, better ways of inviting the life force into my body.
- Planning my financial future. If I have more money than I need. I will work less or give money and things away. I will not think constantly of and work toward a more secure future.
- Thinking about conversations that have not yet happened or have already happened.
- Being around traffic and concrete.

To Increase:
- Sitting in nature.
- Sitting on or holding rocks, to ground me when I must be on technology or indoors.
- Freedom of expression in the way I move my body.
- Girlfriends who embody graceful, flowing feminine energy.
- Art and dance.
- Natural things around me and in the place I live.

- Laughter.
- Children.

I returned from my shamanic journey a different person. After losing my phone, I realized how I had been always thinking in terms of Instagram. *I should get a photo of myself doing this; how will I caption it?"* I thought that it would make me special if people thought I lived an aspirational life. Everything I did had to be documented. I needed my followers to watch. If no one saw me do it, it didn't count. The only reason for doing something was to be recognized for doing it. I had lost my connection to the intrinsic pleasure of being present.

My whole life had been about external validation. I was constantly on the move, working toward my next great achievement; a better body, a higher degree, my own business, bigger waves. My injury tore action and accomplishment away from me. In their place, I found racing thoughts. Without my phone, for the first time in my life, I was moving slow enough, putting enough space between thoughts to actually notice the present moment. Big wave surfing? Sure, if I enjoy it, if I feel up to it, if it makes me feel awesome. But never again would I ride a wave to prove to anybody that I was valuable.

I went almost two months without a phone. It was the best thing besides getting injured that happened to me that year. I became more present in all the things I did. I did many more things for the sake of doing them, for the pleasure inherent in them, than for the recognition I might receive. A huge shift was happening.

At the end of that transformative day, lacking my phone, I made an internet call on my computer to my boyfriend.

"I miss you like crazy. Can you come to Mexico?"

"That's exactly what I want to do!" He was ecstatic.

This man loved me, and I had no idea how to receive that kind of love sexually. We would have to discuss our sex life when he arrived since it was a major factor in our breakup. I didn't know how to associate sex with love. To me, sex was about letting myself be used for pleasure and using other people for validation. Loving sex was an oxymoron. The only way I could feel stimulated sexually was to have that energy brutally stirred up within me--through ramming, taking, and other powerful physical sensations. I had lost my sensitivity to sexual love. But that day, my eyes had been opened to it. I knew the shift would not happen overnight, but it had already begun.

"I want to try again," I told him. I explained that he would need to bring his highest self. I would not tolerate smoking, drinking, or being indoors and zoning out to a screen during daylight hours. He absolutely agreed with me. He said he never wanted to do those things again. And like I had done so many times before, I chose to believe him.

Chapter 39: The Dark Night of the Soul

I was running out the door to complete a last-minute errand before my boyfriend arrived in Mexico. The tile stairs were wet. I slipped, ever so slightly, before regaining balance. On any other day, I would not have noticed the slip, it was so small. But today was special. A familiar hot pain tore through my back. I doubled over and could not straighten back up. Tears filled my eyes. The pain was intense, worse than any of the previous incidents of injury. I knew in an instant that I had re-injured myself worse than all the times before.

For the next several days, I remained bent over, having to crawl to the bathroom and pee in the shower because using the toilet hurt too much. After ten months of solid recovery, the slightest slip on wet tile had set me back farther than ever. The mental pain was worse than the physical. I wasn't getting better; I was getting worse. I knew the next month would be hell on earth. I refused to give in to negative thoughts. I turned back to meditation. I knew I held the power to make this better or worse. The physical suffering was enough. I wasn't going to add mental anguish on top of it. Apparently, I had not yet learned the entirety of the lesson this pain was here to gift me.

For pain, I had been using a powerful Asian herb with opioid-like effects. It was the only thing keeping me sane. Running dangerously low and unable to purchase more in Mexico, I visited every pharmacy in the city with my boyfriend, but we were unable to secure any prescription strength pain medication. Prescription opiates were not available there, and OTC medication did not touch the pain.

With the remaining herbal medication, my condition was tolerable. The medication blocked all the pain receptors in my brain, so although I was uncomfortable, I was still able to show my man around to all my favorite surf spots. We were on another epic adventure, despite the fact that I was taking photos on the beach rather than paddling out. I spent hours laying with my back on the hot sand, visualizing that black energy being sucked from me while he surfed. Things were phenomenal between us. He quit smoking and drinking cold turkey. With the pressure off of sex, it was better than ever. We were connecting on a level I had never known with another human. For days, we surfed and laughed and laid around reading spiritual texts out loud to each other. There were barrels and tacos and orgasms. I didn't know I could be so satisfied without surfing or projects, and while still in pain.

We traveled to the cliffside where I had passed the days immediately following the earthquake. One day while he was surfing I swam out to the line up to meet him. The waves were small and he was surfing the inside point making the swim short and tolerable. I told him I wanted to catch a wave. I hadn't stood up on a surfboard for over six months. Just as I rolled onto his board a waist-high wave came directly toward me. He gave my board a little push. Instinct took over and I felt myself rising to my feet. The wave walled up in front of me. I gave the board a little pump, generating speed. I let the board drop to the bottom trough, crouching low, touching the face of the wave. Then I unloaded the weight from my knees, angling the board toward the lip of the wave. Bottom turn completed, I felt the nose rise over the lip as I straightened out my back leg, pushing with my heal to complete the snap to angle my board back down the face. I looked ahead of me and saw another 100 yards of carvable face. I completed three more turns before hitting the sand still standing on the board. I gently hopped off, pick up the board, and walked back up the beach to my stunned boyfriend, he had never seen me surf before. Some waves are just waves, you ride them and then they are over. Other's leave their mark on you. That wave I will never forget.

We swam naked in a craig between two cliffs that afternoon.
We heard voices calling to us even though no one was around.
We slept under a lonely open-air basilical with a painting of
Mother Mary on the roof. A tropical storm arose that night.
Each strike of lightning illuminated her praying hands. We
were drenched by the early morning hours and retreated to
the car for safety from the lightning strikes all around us. The
next morning we moved on to a new surf spot. Over the next
two weeks, we enjoyed a few other little known sand bottom
point breaks. I paddled out once or twice but couldn't find the
courage to take any waves since the swell had come up.

For the last week of our-month-long Mexican tour, we
returned together to the island I was living on when I learned
I would have to forfeit all of my worldly possessions back in
San Diego. We rented the only decent room on the island. But,
after three days, someone else had a reservation for the room.
We had to find another place to stay. My pain-killing herbs
ran out that day.

We moved into a cabaña equipped with a leaking palapa roof
crawling with spiders and a thick cloud of mosquitoes. There
was a concrete floor and a wooden bed, no toilet seat on the
toilet, and the mattress must have been older than me. My
pain was constant and intense. The shower was just a trickle
of water coming from the wall, right next to a toilet which
may still have had the morning's deposit marinating in it,
depending on whether the toilet decided to flush that day. I
was out of drugs, in the worst pain of my life.

I could not leave the island early because that required a one
hour, bumpy boat ride and a two- hour car ride just to reach
the airport. Then we would need to take at least two flights to
make it to doctors in the States. I had only one defense: my

mind. I was going to stay present through this, no matter how hard it got, because the only other option was suicide. Which did enter my thoughts, repeatedly.

The word "stop" became my best friend. My thoughts ran like crazy. *What if I never recover? What if I will be in this pain for the rest of my life? What if he isn't the right partner for me? What if he goes back to drinking and smoking and TV watching? What will I do with my life to find purpose and meaning? What will I do for money if my body doesn't recover?* STOP!

The most comfortable place to try to relax was a hammock. I found some shade and he strung mine up. I re-focused my attention on the sound of the birds, the glistening of the sun off the ocean, the satisfying feeling of my breath in my lungs. I repurposed the discomfort in my body as a trigger for coming back to the present moment. Each time a spasm shot through my body, I took several deep breaths and moved back into the present.

For hours on end, through sleepless nights and hot, sticky days, I breathed and meditated. *Breathing in, I feel my pain, breathing out I relax into it. Breathing in, I am grateful, breathing out, I am present.* I spent as much time laying on the beach each day as I could tolerate. I let the sun, the sand, and the saltwater pull the darkness from me. Each day required a complete presence of mind. No phones, no computers, no drugs, no cars, no concrete, and, on many days, even no electricity. Just the rise and fall of my lungs, and my supportive partner, who rubbed my feet and reminded me over and over, "You can do this." The pain became so intense that I could not tolerate food. Looking back, I believe the intense suffering caused ulcers. Any food gave me awful cramps and heartburn.

As strange as it sounds, the only way to tolerate the pain was to focus on it. The moment my mind wandered, I was plunged back into torment. Every moment of my day was spent in mindfulness. Breathing and smiling, crying, and accepting, each day I felt a fraction better. After a week, I was well enough to travel. But that week had changed me. I perceived that the true cause of human suffering is not our external circumstances, but the madness of the untrained mind. I had been to the darkest depths, without alcohol, weed, painkillers, coffee, a comfortable bed, reliable shelter, or even very much food. And I had walked out the other side. I had known since my first injury that everything about my life had to change, but now I saw specifically what it was that needed changing. I needed to live in the present moment--and outside of my thoughts. And I had just been given the ultimate test to see if I could do so. Apparently, I was still a straight A student after all as I had passed the most difficult test of my life.

The future holds the promise of success and recognition and popularity and money and security. My mind says I need those things to be happy. But just like I had with dieting, I discovered that I never really wanted to be thin, but to be happy. Happiness, it turned out, was a choice that has nothing to do with circumstances.

Chapter 40: So What Comes Next?

I returned to Hawaii. As soon as the pain was manageable, I got right back to work. Something felt different. As always, I enjoyed doing bodywork. I also enjoyed giving the men a release, seeing all that pent up energy flow out of them. But their gripping, the way they craved me, their compliments...it all drained me rather than filling me.

One day, I was lost in my body work when the client asked me what I was thinking.

"Thinking? I'm not," I replied.

"Oh, come on. You must be thinking something."

I knew what he was after, and it annoyed me. He wanted to know if he was turning me on. Some men just come for their therapy, to relax and receive, knowing that they have paid a fair price in exchange for my touch. But others come for validation. They touch me in ways that are intended to turn me on. They complement my body. They ask how their size compares (and only guys with big dicks ever ask that question; they just want to hear me say it). They think they are going to get me off.

Formerly, my neediness fed off theirs. I hung on every compliment. I craved their hungry touch. My ego soared when they grew ravenous for me. I knew exactly who held the power. The sinful second-class female felt dominate at last.

But things were different now. I wanted to help them. I had great compassion for them. I enjoyed sharing my healing touch with them, connecting with their bodies in an intimate way. But I became annoyed when the needy ones wanted to use me for their own validation. I no longer needed theirs.

"I'm really not thinking anything. I'm feeling. Much of what I'm feeling cannot be described by language. I try not to think. It limits my connection to you and to the work I'm doing."

My response surprised even me. It was true. I had shut down the verbal centers of my brain. I was simply present. Months of meditation and mindfulness training were becoming unconscious habits. My mind was falling quiet. I felt no attraction to the man, and he was clearly disappointed. But I was unwilling to fake it. And I was even willing to give up some power for the sake of dignity.

The money I earned didn't seem important anymore. If my boyfriend was home, I wanted to spend time with him. I turned down hundreds of dollars daily in order to hang out with him or go surfing. I felt the same rebelliousness as I had when I was tired of working at the yoga studio: *none of this matters.*

I no longer posted to Instagram. My followers were dropping away by the day and that was just fine with me. I was relieved not to have to keep up an image. I was hardly surfing since I was still recovering slowly. I surfed only when the waves were small and perfect, and even then just for very short sessions. But my surfs were more enjoyable than ever. My drive to conquer big waves had faded. I still hoped to feel that adrenaline rush again one day, when I was strong once more. But, for now, I was content just to get into the ocean. I was unable to exercise much because of lingering pain, so there was no work towards sculpting a better body. It felt nice to just eat when I was hungry. Another ten pounds had fallen off, and I hovered effortlessly at my high school weight. I had plenty of money to pay bills and buy things I wanted. If I wanted a new car or new clothes, I just accepted a few more appointments. If I wanted to lay on the beach I turned my work phone off. And I was pretty much content. As long as I kept up with my meditation practice and worked hard to keep my thoughts in check, I felt pretty good.

They had promised me that if I checked all the boxes that I would live happily ever after. Good grades, college education, marriage, house, kids. I tried it their way - two marriages and college degrees and good jobs. And I was not happy. So I tried it another way. I went on my traveling adventure, had my flings, and took my risks, prizing my beauty, athleticism, and my rebelliousness. I went looking for the edge until I found it and leapt off it. And it all made me happy. So happy. But not *happily ever after*. Happy at that moment.

Now, the moment had passed. I was content, yes. And out of that contentment, I sensed a lingering desire for a new challenge. It seemed just around the corner. What's next? I knew it would not be a challenge that I would accept in order to set myself up for the future or to endear myself to others. Whatever drama lay before me would unfold for only one reason, to bring me more deeply into the present.

I've surfed waves bigger than houses and suffered the consequences. I left a drug addict husband when I was penniless. I abandoned everything I owned and drove alone through cartel-run drug territory in Mexico. I had my fingers down my throat for three years straight. I endured the most intense physical pain. And I needed every minute of these challenges. I would not have traded any of it. I was the person I was because of these experiences. And I loved who I was. And now, the next great challenge stirred within me. What new rebirth lay ahead?

I wanted a challenge that would make me reach within for my deepest goodness. I wanted to find my highest, purest self. I wanted to trim off all the remaining fat.

I had been bouncing around the globe for three years. Nine new stamps adorned my passport. I had become bilingual. All my possessions fit in one car. I had an amazing partner. I had a healthy body at a stable weight, a mostly positive body image, and sufficient money. I asked the universe to reveal its next gift.

I knew the next phase would change my life even more. I knew my life would never again be about what Natasha could accomplish. I knew better than to think the challenge would fulfill me or give me a lasting sense of purpose. I wanted a new experience, just to experience it. I wanted to be stretched and expanded. I wanted the next big wave to come and teach me even more about what it means to be alive. I wanted to be pulled even deeper into the perfection of my humanity. The challenge wouldn't be about accomplishing; it would be about uncovering.

Some say surfing is the most challenging and rewarding endeavor you will ever undertake. It is so hard that even a simple turn is considered an advanced maneuver. It is so frustrating because the progress is painfully slow, and there seem to be more failures than successes. It is so slow that you don't notice progress happening at all. Then, one day you look up and you are staring out of a barrel. And, well, I don't know of any feeling more rewarding than knowing you teamed up with the power and flow of nature and she deemed you worthy to come inside.

The reality was that my progress in surfing may forever have been at a halt. I could learn to enjoy it more. But, with the state of my body, I likely would not become significantly more proficient in my lifetime. Humans are made to spend their lives uncovering their most authentic selves. Not for the photos or awards or outside validation, but for the intrinsic pleasure of doing something you love with intense focus and enjoyment. I wondered what that something would be.

Then, one day while at my physical therapist's office I glanced in the mirror to check my form. I was startled by how large my breast appeared. They had been aching and I assumed it was because I would get my period any day now. When I got home I peed on a stick, like I've done a dozen times before. I was certain the result would be like all the times before. But this time two lines appeared. Ohmygod, ohmygod, I'm going to be a mother!

He held me as I wept. Wildly different emotions consumed me, all at once. Pure excitement, sheer terror. I wanted to turn back. We had said we wanted to try to get pregnant. We tried exactly one time and then, apprehensive, we decided to go back to using preventative measures. And now it was like a payment had been submitted before I'd clicked Confirm. *What have I done? What if I hate being a mom? What if I miss my freedom?* At the same time, my heart soared. Even though I had no idea what was coming for me, I knew it was exactly what I wanted. I invited this soul to come be my teacher, and it agreed. I couldn't even imagine where we would go.

Fear followed on the heels of euphoria. How would I provide for this child? My partner had just lost his job, and I knew I couldn't do sensual massage with a big belly and leaking boobs. *I don't want to go back to working a job I don't like. I don't want to be a working mom with a little baby. I don't want to be scared about how the rent will get paid.* The racing thoughts were back. Already, the challenge of motherhood was homing in on my growth areas. Flowing with nature? Apparently, there was much work still to be done.

How ironic. I still don't fully trust in the ultimate goodness of the universe. With all the lessons I have already learned, I still have to work on flow. Here is my work to do, right here, growing in my belly.

Life is like that. It doesn't get any easier. It just gets more real. I get closer and closer to my true self. Each new chapter in my life has marked the casting off of some ego that I wore as a mask so people would love me. A few months from now, I will be as vulnerable and real as it gets. Laying naked, legs spread wide, grunting and moaning with pain and bliss. Will I trust my truest self in that moment? Is there a woman inside who is the source of life itself? Is this body truly a miracle worker, a divinely powered structure? Does the divine wisdom that now knits my child together within my womb also have permission to run my life? Will I surrender to who I already am?

They promised me motherhood would be happily ever after. I know it's a lie. Motherhood is going to be the same as marriage or road trips or surfing or eating or sex. Happiness is a choice, made in each new moment. It exists nowhere in the future. So here I go, marching boldly into the next great adventure, where I will find happiness along with every other emotion of the human spectrum. But this is what I was made for. Onward and inward, sweet soul.

Chapter 41: My Story

An idea came to me in a whirlwind. I was staring off into the waves when a voice spoke inside my head. "Tell your story," it said. "Tell the story of Natash Black, a sacred sexual healer, a soul surfer, a mother. Tell it because you want *it* to be heard, not because *you* want to be heard. Tell it because the telling will give you joy. Tell it because one person might relate. Tell it so you don't forget and so you keep growing."

A book about sex work and all my triumphs and struggles, under a pen name? A book where I'll never receive any personal recognition or fame? A book about who I really am, in which I don't have to convince anyone to like me? A space where I don't have to give a fuck if I'm fat or thin or if I surf big waves or if I have a lot of followers? That book could be the beginning of a space in this world where I can be completely who I am, hiding nothing of myself, owing nothing to anyone, proving nothing about my worthiness. In that space, I hold the power of self-approval. The power is not in the hands of my followers, my partner, men, my mother, or even my readers.

I can't write down the answers to an eating disorder or fragmented self-esteem or years of religious abuse. But I can uncover it within myself. This book is the experience of knowing. A kind of knowing that cannot be taught, but only experienced. Dear reader, thank you for having this experience with me.

Afterword

Eleven weeks ago I inhabited my body more than ever before. I thought birth would be surreal, an out of body experience where, once again, my mind would have control over my body. It was nothing of the sort. My body was going to do anything it had to, up to and including killing me, in order to bring my son into this world. In the final moments of my unmedicated birth I became one with all that is. The power of all of nature filled my body as I let go of any scraps of ego that remained. I became a vessel, a tool created by nature for growing human life. I wasn't a big wave surfer or sexy woman or straight A daughter. I was Force, I was life itself. And at the same time I was just a part of evolution, doomed to the same fate as all creatures in the cycle of life. A sound I've never heard came from deep within me. My partner said later that the walls shook. Some unknown force took over my body as it tore itself apart from the inside out. And then, then I saw my son for the very first time.

I type this with one hand while I hold my son's head to my breast with the other. I invited this soul into my life to be my teacher. I was put on this earth to have an experience. Each experience is here to help me workout some karmic debt. I chose to have big experiences, to learn big lessons. This is a big thing. From my body and love I made life. Sweet salvation from my own veins dreams next to me now. I now snuggle up to an innocent baby sent to save me, break me open, change me-- this perfect, loud child. I was once a student of the ocean. Now I lose myself in his waters.

But salvation doesn't mean that the facedown on the bathroom floor in a puddle of my own snot and tears moments have ended. In fact They seem to be increasing in frequency. Just last month I found myself in that familiar messy heap because my partner and I don't feel all the warm and fuzzies we did when we decided to make this perfect creation. Running on very little sleep, disagreeing about parenting techniques and sleeping in different rooms so someone can get a few hours of rest. I feel like I'm walking on eggshells. Everything I say puts distance between us. Everything he doesn't say brings hot tears to my eyes. I guess I was still using the power that sex brought me to control my partner. Now with very few opportunities for sex and a partner that is to sure of himself to be controlled I find myself miserable once again. It's too hard, too hard. Did I pick the wrong partner? Is this my own issue of worthiness? And once again the sound track in my head starts up louder than ever.

It doesn't get better. Or, it does and it doesn't. Life is just life. It's made up of a million trillion little moments of looking out of barrels, of hearts connecting at an atomic level--and of flat tires on the freeway and washing vomit from my face. I'm searching for my box. I want to put a bow on this whole saga, to close it all up for you in a neat package. I want to find some truth and to say I lived happily ever after.

Or maybe my urge to end this with some great moral teaching, like the final line in an Aesop's' Fable, is because I need to convince myself, more than anyone, that something redemptive happened to me, that I found salvation. I'd love to draw the silver thread of truth through the last 41 chapters. *I once was lost but now I'm found. Amazing grace saved a wretch like me.*

I doubt there really is such a thing as salvation. Maybe we are forever and continuously being saved-- now, here, right now, where I'm writing this. I stare into the perfect face of my son. His body seems to melt into mine. Out my front window, the surf is pumping but I can't move because he will wake up. Every couple of minutes he stirs in his sleep. He wants to re-latch onto my breast. He starts to suckle. Oxytocin floods my brain and suddenly the love I feel for this tiny being is stronger than the ocean.

Perhaps the moral of the story is that there is no salvation because I never needed saving. I was never lost because there is no destination to find, nor is there a journey. So I guess this story doesn't end happily ever. I'll just go on living, sometimes happy, sometimes not, but always present, always saved.

Natasha Black is a surfer, writer and mom who lives in an
undisclosed surfing paradise. Follower her blog *Salt and Sugar*
at NatashaBlackAuthor.com